Comments from readers:

'I think [this book] is excellently compiled.'

TIM HILLARD,
Consultant Obstetrician and Gynaecologist

'As an expert on herbal medicines used by many as an alternative to HRT, I consider that Dr Currie's analysis is fair, balanced and accurate.'

Professor EDZARD ERNST, MD, PhD, FRCP, FRCP (Edin.),
Professor of Complementary Medicine, Peninsula Medical School, UK

'Finding that [symptoms] are part of the menopause and that you are not going mad, can be very helpful!'

SARAH GRAY, GP (Truro),
Adviser to NICE

'All in all, it is undoubtedly the best and certainly the most sensible book I've yet to read on the subject.'

VAL HIRST, *Newark*

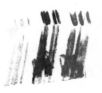

Menopause

Answers at your fingertips

Dr Heather Currie MB, BS, FRCOG, MRCGP, MFFP

Associate Specialist Gynaecologist and Obstetrician
Dumfries and Galloway Royal Infirmary, Dumfries
Managing Director of Menopause Matters Ltd

with a chapter by

Sister Katrina Martin BSc, RGN

Specialist Menopause and Osteoporosis Nurse
Dumfries and Galloway Royal Infirmary, Dumfries

CLASS PUBLISHING • LONDON

Printing history
First published 2006

The author and publishers welcome feedback from the users of this book.
Please contact the publishers.

**Class Publishing, Barb House, Barb Mews, London W6 7PA, UK
Telephone: 020 7371 2119 / Fax: 020 7371 2878 [International +4420]
email: post@class.co.uk / website: www.class.co.uk**

The information presented in this book is accurate and current to the best
of the author's knowledge. The author and publisher, however, make no
guarantee as to, and assume no responsibility for, the correctness, sufficiency
or completeness of such information or recommendation. The reader is
advised to consult a doctor regarding all aspects of individual healthcare.

A CIP catalogue record for this book is available from the British Library

ISBN 10 1859591558

ISBN 13 9781859591550

10 9   8   7   6   5   4   3   2   1

Edited and indexed by Michèle Clarke

Designed and typeset by Martin Bristow

Artwork by David Woodroffe

Cartoons by Jane Taylor

Printed and bound in Finland by WS Bookwell, Juva

Contents

Foreword

The menopause is a natural event. It is also inevitable – all women who live long enough will experience it. Some will hardly notice it; others will suffer troublesome symptoms, occasionally lasting for months or even years. For many, it represents a time of change; a time when fertility stops and hormones can play havoc with your emotions. With up to 75% of women in the UK experiencing physical symptoms, it is bad enough, but when you start to feel as if you are going mad it really is time to seek help!

This book seeks to answer all those questions you have been afraid to ask, all those issues that seem trivial but which, when answered, put your mind at rest. You wonder what is normal, what you should be experiencing and how you might help yourself through the symptoms. What treatments are available? Is HRT safe? What exactly is HRT anyway? Is there anything else I can take? Then you want to know about your long-term health – what measures can you take to keep healthy, how will the hormonal changes affect your future health?

Written by an expert menopause practitioner, this book answers all these questions and many more in a way that is relevant to women and easy to understand. You will dip into it time and time again.

Kathy Abernethy
Senior Nurse Specialist
The Menopause Clinical and Research Unit
Northwick Park Hospital, Harrow, Middlesex

Acknowledgements

I should like to thank Kathy Abernethy, Julie Ayres, Professor Ernst, Ailsa Gebbie, Sarah Gray, Tim Hillard and Val Hirst for their diligent and very helpful reviews; Dr Jane Johnston for her input with the chapter on alternative and complementary therapies; Michèle Clarke for her outstanding editorial skills; and finally my colleagues at work, both past and present, for their support.

To Matthew, Victoria, James, the rest of my family and my friends
for their encouragement, patience and endless support,
and for giving me the confidence to 'give it a go'.

Introduction

The menopause is important and can have significant consequences, but should not be dreaded as a serious illness; it is another phase in the rich tapestry of a woman's hormonal life!

The menopause and its treatment, and indeed whether or not it should be treated at all, continues to be controversial with many diverse opinions frequently being discussed. Both women and their doctors are often very confused about which is the right course of action. To reduce this confusion, it is essential that any woman has access to accurate information about what happens at the menopause, what the effects can be, what treatments are available and, not least, what she can do herself to live life as healthily and fully as possible. This book aims to provide such information in a detailed, yet readable form.

In each chapter, comprehensive information about the topic is backed up by real questions and answers – questions that are important yet are rarely covered in standard text books. The book can be read from start to finish, or you may want to just read certain chapters relevant to the stage that you are in currently. For example, you may not yet be having menopausal problems and simply want to find out why and when the menopause occurs so as to be prepared, but at a later date you may want to know more about the symptoms and treatment options. For further information, an extensive resources section includes details of support organisations, helplines, websites and other books.

We are sure that you will find this book useful, enjoyable and inspiring!

Note to reader
There is a glossary at the end of this book to help you with any words that may be unfamiliar to you (printed in *italics* in the text). If you are looking for particular topics, you can use either the detailed list of Contents or the Index.

1 | The menopause – what happens and when?

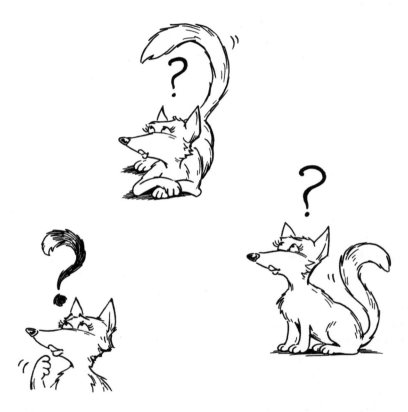

Love it or loathe it, the menopause affects all women worldwide, although attitudes towards the menopause vary between different cultures. In some, the menopause is seen very negatively as the end of fertility and lowering of status compared with younger, fertile, beautiful women; yet in others, it is celebrated as the end of monthly impurity and restrictions from taboos, with the beginning of an age of maturity, wisdom and freedom. In countries such as India where the menopause is viewed positively, drug treatment for the menopause is minimal. Attitudes towards the menopause across cultures are affected by environments, diets, climate, lifestyle, religion, taboos and genetics.

For most women, it occurs naturally, when the *ovaries* spontaneously fail to produce the all-important hormones, *oestrogen* and *progesterone*. For some women, ovaries stop working owing to specific treatment such as chemotherapy or radiotherapy, or the menopause may occur after the ovaries have been removed, often at the time of a *hysterectomy* (removal of the womb).

What does the word 'menopause' actually mean?

Menopause means the 'last menstrual period'. It is derived from the Greek word 'menos', meaning a month, and 'pausos', an ending. Periods stop because the low levels of oestrogen and progesterone do not stimulate the lining of the womb in the normal cycle. These hormones and their fluctuating levels are described below in **The menstrual cycle**.

The term *climacteric* refers to the time in which the hormone levels are changing, up to when the periods stop; lowering and fluctuating hormone levels can cause early menopausal symptoms while still stimulating the lining of the womb to produce cyclical bleeding (*menstruation*).

Perimenopause is the stage from the beginning of menopausal symptoms to the post-menopause. *Post-menopause* is the time following the last period, and this is usually defined as more than 12 months with no periods in someone with intact ovaries, or immediately following surgery if the ovaries have been removed.

THE MENSTRUAL CYCLE

To understand what happens at the menopause stage and the changes leading up to the menopause, it is important to understand the normal *menstrual cycle* (Fig. 1.1). For ovaries to function, a complex interaction occurs between the *pituitary gland* (at the base of the brain), egg cells within the ovaries responding to chemical stimulation, and the release of hormones from the ovaries.

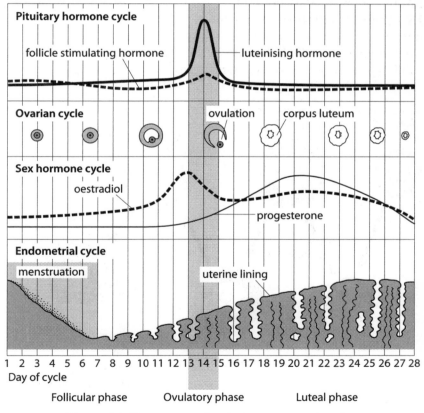

Figure 1.1 Hormone cycles during menstrual cycles.

Follicular phase

The first day of a period is called day 1 of the menstrual cycle. In the few days leading up to day 1, if pregnancy has not occurred, oestrogen and progesterone levels fall and this fall leads to a shedding of the lining of the womb – *menstruation*. The fall in oestrogen and *inhibin* (a hormone which has been researched only fairly recently), also allows a rise in *follicle stimulating hormone (FSH)*, which is produced from the pituitary gland, since high levels of oestrogen and inhibin suppress FSH production through a feedback mechanism. FSH then stimulates development of follicles in the ovary and, by days 5 to 7, usually one follicle in particular continues to respond. This 'dominant' follicle produces large amounts of oestrogen and inhibin from its granulosa cells, resulting in a fall in FSH.

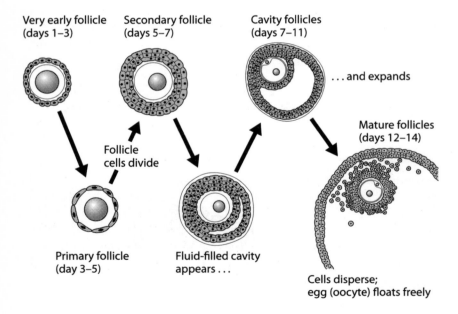

Figure 1.2 Follicle.

Other effects of oestrogen at this stage include stimulation of the lining of the womb to become thickened, ready to receive a fertilised egg.

Ovulatory phase

At about days 12 to 14, high oestrogen levels stimulate release of *luteinising hormone (LH)* from the pituitary gland. The surge in LH causes the egg to be released from the follicle (*ovulation*).

Luteal phase

During days 14 to 28, the area of the ovary that has released the egg, the *corpus luteum*, produces progesterone. Progesterone further prepares the womb lining for accepting a fertilised egg. If the egg is not fertilised, the corpus luteum 'collapses' and the levels of oestrogen and progesterone fall. Without these hormones to support the lining, the womb then sheds its lining and menstruation begins again. Also, with a low oestrogen level, FSH rises and a new cycle begins.

So what happens to this cycle leading up to and during the menopause?

The maximum number of egg cells (oocytes) within the ovaries is present before you are born; by about the fifth month of gestation there are thought to be around 7 million, and these decline to 1–2 million by birth. From birth onwards there is a gradual reduction, with about 400,000 remaining by the time of puberty, thereafter a gradual decline by the age of 40 years and then a rapid decline up to the menopause. Leading up to the menopause, the follicles remaining are not only fewer in number but also less able to respond to the stimulation by FSH. Occasionally, cycles occur where follicles have not developed fully and less oestrogen is produced. Low levels of oestrogen lead to menopausal symptoms, a rise in FSH, and a failure to trigger the LH surge leading to absence of ovulation. With no ovulation, progesterone production is also reduced, leading to irregular shedding of the lining of the womb and hence irregular periods. In the early stages, the ovaries fluctuate in how well they work, so that cycles may be normal some months and abnormal in others. Gradually the number of abnormal cycles increases so that eventually, no follicles develop, oestrogen and progesterone production becomes very low, the lining of the womb is not stimulated at all, periods stop and FSH levels remain high.

The low and changing levels of hormones, particularly oestrogen, are thought to be the cause of menopausal symptoms (see Chapter 3) in many women.

Some doctors think that many of the changes occurring at the menopause because of the falling hormone levels can be thought of as the results of the body's poor adaptation to the same falling hormone levels that occur following childbirth.

- An increase in your body heat is helpful following childbirth in order to warm the baby, but this effect during the menopause causes hot flushes.

- A poor sleep pattern maintains vigilance for the baby, but later leads to insomnia and subsequent tiredness.

- Getting the calcium from your bones is important to provide calcium for the baby through your breast milk, but can later cause you to develop osteoporosis.

- High blood levels of fat provide calories for the baby through your breast milk, but at the menopause can lead to fatty deposits in your arteries and atherosclerosis.

The changes during the menopause therefore should be taken seriously and all women should have access to appropriate information and advice to help them manage these changes.

Why did my periods become erratic before they stopped?

In the early stages, the levels of FSH, LH, oestrogen and progesterone fluctuate markedly and symptoms and period patterns may change from month to month. Often the falling progesterone level, which regulates the lining of your womb (the *endometrium*), causes erratic, heavy or prolonged periods before any other menopausal symptoms are noticed. Hormone levels can fluctuate for several years before eventually becoming so low that the endometrium stays thin and does not bleed.

I'm 45 and my periods are awful – sometimes I miss a month and then have the period from hell! Last month I flooded through a super tampon and a pad and stained my friend's cream sofa – I was so embarrassed. Surely this can't be normal?

This pattern happens quite often in the stage leading up to the menopause. Although it is very likely due to changing hormone production, you should discuss the problem with your doctor who might suggest some tests to rule out other causes. Very effective treatments are available and no woman should have to put up with such inconvenience.

My doctor tells me not to worry about my periods being irregular. She says it is because I am perimenopausal, but what does this mean?

Perimenopause is the phase when the ovaries are still working and producing hormones but are not producing the correct balance of hormones to stimulate the womb lining to shed regularly. Hence the lining may be shed either more or less often than before, resulting in irregular periods. At this stage you may also notice some menopausal symptoms, since the oestrogen level may be lower than previously.

I am in my late 40s and don't think I have ever had a hot flush, but my periods are increasingly irregular and sometimes heavy. Is this the menopause and how long can I expect it to carry on like this? It's a real nuisance.

As the ovaries gradually decline and produce a different balance of hormones, a change in the pattern of your periods often occurs. This can go on for a number of years before the periods actually stop. The 'menopause' is the final period, so this is not the actual menopause yet but is the stage leading up to the menopause. However, a change in your periods, such as periods becoming more frequent or heavy, or bleeding between periods, should be discussed with your doctor to make sure there is not some other cause. Very effective treatments are available.

I had 3 months when I missed periods and noticed some hot feelings, like my face was burning up. Then my periods came back and the hot feelings went. What was going on?

This often happens before the periods finally stop and is a sign of the ovarian function fluctuating. When the hormone production is low, the periods stop because the endometrium isn't being stimulated and the low levels may cause symptoms like hot flushes. (Read more about symptoms in Chapter 3.) Then, for a while, the ovaries may produce the correct level of hormones again, producing regular bleeds. This fluctuation may continue for a few years before the actual menopause.

WHEN DOES THE MENOPAUSE HAPPEN?

The average age at which the natural menopause occurs is 51 years, but it can happen much earlier or later. This average age varies between different countries: it occurs earlier in southern African women compared with Europeans; it even varies within countries –

it has been found that malnourished women in Papua New Guinea undergo the menopause at an average age of 43.6 years compared with 47.3 years in well-nourished women in the same country, supporting the idea that nutrition affects the age at which the menopause occurs. This age is also affected by smoking: women who smoke become menopausal up to 2 years earlier than non-smokers, perhaps owing to cigarette smoke accelerating ageing of egg cells.

A menopause occurring before the age of 45 is called an 'early menopause', and before the age of 40 it is known as a 'premature menopause'. Premature or early menopause can be a devastating diagnosis, especially if you wanted to have more children. It most often occurs spontaneously, i.e. without any specific reason, or it may follow surgery such as a hysterectomy when the ovaries might be removed along with the womb (*oophorectomy*).

If the ovaries are left in place at the time of hysterectomy, the menopause can still happen early, possibly owing to interference with the blood supply to the ovaries at the time of the operation.

Other causes of early or premature menopause include chromosomal disorders such as Turner's syndrome and Down's syndrome, *autoimmune disorder* (when antibodies that work against the ovaries are produced), and chemotherapy or radiotherapy. Some drugs may stop the ovaries functioning but this usually resumes when the drug is stopped. Women who have chromosomal disorders often do not have periods at all, since their hormone levels will have always been low. They may not experience the usual menopausal symptoms since they do not have changing hormone levels.

Despite the lack of symptoms, discussion about hormonal treatment is vitally important, as it is for all women with premature menopause, since they have an increased risk of *osteoporosis*. Oestrogen is very important in the development and maintenance of strong bones. If a woman is deprived of oestrogen at a younger age than normal, then there is an increased risk of bone thinning, or osteoporosis, which can increase the risk of fracture in later life.

Why was I told to keep taking HRT until I'm 50? I had an early menopause when I was 38.

Generally, women having an early or premature menopause are advised to take HRT until approximately the average age of the menopause, for both symptom control and for its bone-protective effect. Although there is concern about using HRT for long periods, it is generally believed that the risks, particularly of an increase in breast cancer with long-term use, apply to women who take HRT for over 5 years after the age of 50. For young women, as long as there is no medical reason for avoiding HRT, the benefits of taking HRT up to the age of 50 are likely to outweigh the risks. We talk more about HRT in Chapter 8.

I stopped the pill to try to become pregnant but my periods didn't come and I was having terrible hot flushes. After a few months I went to my doctor. He did blood tests and has told me that I'm menopausal. I'm only 31 – I can't believe that I'm having the menopause and can't have any children. I feel as if my world has fallen apart. Could the tests be wrong?

Premature menopause can sometimes be temporary, meaning that the ovaries may start producing eggs and hormones again. As well as checking hormone levels, your GP may take blood tests to see if there is any correctable cause such as high prolactin levels or something wrong with your thyroid function. If there is no apparent underlying cause and you continue not to have any periods, with repeat hormone levels showing menopausal changes, then it is likely that the diagnosis is correct. Although this is difficult to come to terms with, help is available.

- Knowing that you are not alone always helps and there are some excellent support groups for premature menopause (see *Appendix 1*).

- Regarding future fertility, pregnancies have been achieved using egg donation. Although there may be a long waiting list for treatment and, in some areas of the country, fertility treatments have to be paid for, it is definitely worth looking into. Some women have family members who are willing to be donors and this can shorten the waiting time.

- Thirdly, the symptoms of hot flushes can be very effectively treated and, in young women like yourself experiencing the menopause, HRT is usually recommended both to control symptoms and to provide a beneficial effect on bones.

Why am I still l having periods at my age of 55?

Late menopause can occur but, by the age of 54, 80% of women will have stopped having periods because their ovarian function has stopped but 20% continue having periods beyond 54. It is very unusual for periods to continue beyond 58 but the oldest recorded age of a women still having periods is 104! If your periods stop for more than 1 year and then bleeding restarts, go and see your doctor.

My mum became menopausal when she was 35. Is that likely to happen to me?

Often there is no obvious cause of premature or early menopause but there might be a family history of it. There could have been a specific cause for your mum's premature menopause but, if it occurred out of the blue, then you should look out for early signs in yourself, since some women do follow a pattern of menopause at a similar time to their mothers.

2 | Diagnosing the menopause

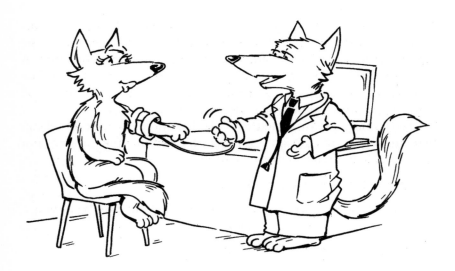

Many women may suspect that the problems they have are due to hormone changes but may not ask for a diagnosis, because they associate the menopause with old age; none of us wants to feel old! However, facing up to the diagnosis can lead to appropriate advice and treatment, allowing you to move forward with help and support when needed. The menopause is another stage; it is not a dreadful illness!

The absence of periods for more than 1 year in a woman in her late 40s or 50s, associated with some menopausal symptoms, is clearly due to the menopause and specific tests are not required. It is often in young women and in the early, perimenopausal years that there may be uncertainty about the cause of symptoms, and tests may then be taken to diagnose whether it really is the menopause.

How is the menopause diagnosed?

With declining function of the ovaries, levels of follicle stimulating hormone (FSH) and luteinising hormone (LH) rise. Measurements of FSH are often used to diagnose the menopause. A diagnosis of the menopause will be made from a combination of factors, with most emphasis being placed on the history of your period pattern and presence of any menopausal symptoms.

Occasionally, measurement of FSH, LH and oestrogen levels can help make the diagnosis but are not essential and usually not required. Measurements are most useful when

- premature menopause is suspected

- there is no period pattern to observe following a hysterectomy without removal of the ovaries

- unusual symptoms are present, or

- fertility appears to be reduced.

I have seen some kits in my local pharmacy for measurement of FSH. Would it be worth getting one?

Home kits can be used to check for a raised FSH level in a urine test, but you can also have a blood test to measure this level; however, the level depends on the phase of your cycle and fluctuates markedly over time. If you do go and have a test, make sure that the blood sample is taken on the 3rd to 5th day of your period. A normal level does not exclude the possibility of an early menopause, and a raised level does not exclude continuing ovarian function.

When my periods stopped, I had a blood test which showed
menopausal hormone levels. I was started on HRT but after
3 months I became pregnant – how could this have happened?

Because hormone levels and ovarian function fluctuate so much, one raised level should not be relied upon as a reason to stop using contraception, since decline of ovarian function can be temporary and egg release can still occur late in your transition to the menopause. None of the currently used HRT preparations is licensed for contraception, so, when you are in the early phase of menopause, you should continue to use contraception if you don't want to become pregnant. (See Chapter 6 for more information on contraception.)

Note that FSH levels can be temporarily raised after the oral contraceptive pill or long acting progestogen contraceptives are stopped, during breast feeding, in severe illness, hypothyroidism, depression, after radiotherapy or chemotherapy, and also with some medicines such as the antidepressant selective serotonin reuptake inhibitors, for example fluoxetine (Prozac).

Should I have other tests at this time?

This stage in your life is a good time to consider your general health and fitness by having your blood pressure and weight measured. You should also think about your exercise levels, diet, smoking and alcohol intake (see Chapter 7).

Blood tests could include one for *thyroid function*, since thyroid disorder is very common and can often cause similar symptoms to the menopause. Other tests such as a full hormone profile, including prolactin level, and occasionally *chromosome analysis*, should be considered only if the menopause is premature.

3 | Menopause symptoms

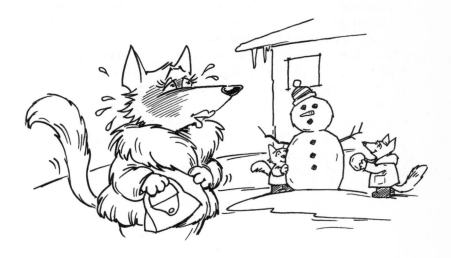

Menopausal symptoms, which affect about 70–80% of women, are believed to be due to the changing hormone levels, particularly oestrogen, but many factors such as *diet, exercise and lifestyle* (see Chapter 7), and other *medications* or *medical problems* (see Chapter 11) can influence the symptoms. Therefore, for some people, lifestyle factors such as reducing/stopping smoking, reducing alcohol and caffeine intake, reducing stress, eating healthily and taking regular exercise can considerably help the symptoms of menopause.

For others, HRT can be very beneficial, and indeed menopausal symptom control is the main indication for using HRT. If you are prescribed HRT to relieve symptoms like these, and for no other reason, your doctor is likely to recommend you stop taking it every 2 years or so to find out whether you still need treatment. If you find that your symptoms come back when you do stop, talk to your doctor about starting to take it again. It may well be that, for you, the benefits will outweigh the risks (see Chapter 8).

Many women choose to try *alternative or complementary therapies* to control the symptoms of their menopause (see Chapter 10). Talking to others about symptoms or joining a support group to be reassured that you are not alone can impart a huge benefit to your psychological welfare. Symptoms may cause extra worry – you may think that they are due to some other potentially serious illness. Finding that they are part of the menopause and that you are not going mad, can be very helpful!

Menopausal symptoms affect cultures differently and cultural influences have an effect on coping mechanisms: in Japan, hot flushes, sweats and poor sleeping seem to be less common than in western cultures, but headaches are a common menopausal symptom. Also in Japan, hot flushes are regarded as a 'luxury disease' for women who have too much spare time and are selfish! It is possible that this attitude would deter reporting of such symptoms. In India, hot flushes are not known but it is unclear whether they really are absent or are perceived differently. In some cultures the term 'hot flush' is not translatable so asking about hot flushes may produce a negative response. However, questions can be phrased differently, and in another culture women may be asked, 'Are you on fire?'

I am 47 and have noticed what I presume are menopausal symptoms. When do menopausal symptoms normally begin?

Many women notice early symptoms while they are still having periods, when the hormone production is declining very gradually. This stage of gradually falling and fluctuating hormone levels is often called the *climacteric* or the 'change' and it often begins in the 40s – it can last for several years. Because ovarian function fluctuates, women may experience symptoms intermittently. Some women experience an early, or premature menopause following which symptoms may occur immediately, depending on the cause.

Immediate onset of menopause symptoms often follows a *surgical menopause* when the ovaries are removed at an operation (see Chapter 5).

WHAT ARE THE SYMPTOMS OF THE MENOPAUSE?

Early menopause symptoms include physical, psychological and sexual problems.

Physical symptoms

Physical symptoms include:

- hot flushes
- night sweats
- palpitations
- insomnia
- joint aches
- weight gain
- breast tenderness
- headaches.

Hot flushes

The hot flush, or flash, is well known as the classic menopausal symptom and affects 60–85% of menopausal women. Hot flushes and sweats are called *vasomotor symptoms* and vary immensely in both their severity and duration; for many women, they occur occasionally and do not cause much distress, but for about 20% they can be severe and can cause significant interference with work, sleep and quality of life. Women are affected by vasomotor symptoms on average for about 2 years but, for about 10%, symptoms can continue for more than 15 years.

During a flush, your upper body, arms and face feel hot, your skin turns red, and sweating may occur. Some women experience total body heat, may drip in sweat and may wake up several times a night drenched in sweat. Hot flushes usually last 3–5 minutes and are thought to be caused by a change in the temperature-controlling part of the brain. If you have an infection, your body temperature may rise. When it rises above a critical level, you start sweating and this helps to cool you down. Similarly, if the body temperature falls below a critical level, mechanisms occur whereby the body shivers and the body heats up.

Symptomatic menopausal women flush, sweat and sometimes feel cold with much smaller changes in body temperature. Normally, there is a daily pattern of rises and falls in your body temperature, being lowest at about 3am and highest in the early evening. These small changes are not normally noticed, but a menopausal woman may flush with every temperature rise, whether these are normal changes or not – for example, moving between areas of different temperature or having a hot drink – because of a change in the setting of the temperature control centre in your brain; your body thinks that it is overheating even when it isn't. To try to cool your body down, a variety of chemical reactions cause the blood vessels in the skin to open up, giving the sensation of a rush of heat, and sweat glands release sweat to dissipate heat.

It is believed that the changes in various hormone levels that occur around the time of the menopause, lead to the change in the setting of the temperature control centre, but the exact underlying mechanism is still unclear.

Recent research has proposed that there is normally a neutral temperature zone in which small changes in temperature do not trigger either cooling down or heating up mechanisms; it is a 'buffering zone', which allows the body to cope with variations in temperature. Menopausal women who have vasomotor symptoms appear to have a much reduced 'buffering zone' so that small changes in temperature trigger the cooling down or heating up mechanisms. What is still unclear is what causes some women to develop this reduced zone and why some menopausal women maintain the normal zone and hence do not have flushes.

The low and changing level of the hormone oestrogen is very important in temperature control and the replacement of oestrogen in HRT is the most effective treatment for menopausal symptoms. Oestrogen is thought to raise the setting of the temperature control back to its normal level. Other chemicals such as serotonin, gamma-aminobutyric acid and noradrenaline have also been shown to be involved in temperature control. When doctors realised that non-hormonal chemicals also have effects, this led to the use of treatments for vasomotor symptoms other than HRT, both prescribed and alternative therapies, but further research is ongoing.

Other factors that can also cause flushes include being overweight, alcohol, excess caffeine, spicy foods, monosodium glutamate and some medications. Eating a healthy diet and losing weight if necessary can be helpful. Other simple measures that can help include:

- wearing cotton clothing rather than man-made fibres

- wearing loose thin layers of clothing rather than thick tight-fitting clothes

- keeping your bedroom temperature fairly cool at night – either leave a door or window open or consider a fan (partner permitting of course!).

Flushes affect every woman differently and, for many, no specific treatments will be required. When flushes are embarrassing, disruptive and affecting your quality of life, then help is available and your doctor will give you an individualised treatment plan – we are all unique!

Headaches, palpitations (sensation of heart racing) and dizziness can be associated with vasomotor symptoms. Excess caffeine can worsen palpitations, so take coffee, tea and caffeinated soft drinks in moderation.

What is the best way to cope with getting hot flushes in the office? I get particularly worried when I am attending important board meetings and things like that.

Specific treatments can be used to control hot flushes but, if you prefer to cope without treatment, then simple measures such as wearing thin layers of clothing instead of thick clothes, not sitting next to a heater, reducing hot drinks, and not worrying about it can help – stress can increase flushes so the more you worry that you are going to have one, the more likely it is that you will!

Sleeplessness

I have hot flushes – they don't really bother me – the worst thing is not sleeping. I can be absolutely exhausted when I go to bed and I go off to sleep OK, but then I wake up at any time between 2 and 4am. I then toss and turn and eventually get back to sleep but it only seems a short while later when the alarm goes off. I long for a full night's sleep. What can I do?

Insomnia (sleeplessness) or disturbed sleep (leading to tiredness and fatigue), may be partly due to the night sweats, control of which can lead to an improved sleep pattern, but insomnia has also been shown to be a menopausal symptom regardless of the presence of temperature changes and may begin a few years before the menopause.

Simple measures such as taking time to relax before going to bed by reading, watching television, or having a bath can make sure that you're not going to bed with your brain working overtime! Try to avoid caffeine or nicotine for at least 4 hours before bed time and don't have the bedroom too hot. Exercise during the day can help but don't exercise just before going to bed. Sometimes it actually helps to get up for a while, since lying and thinking about getting to sleep can make it harder to go off.

HRT has been shown to reduce insomnia and, because of the disruptive knock-on effects of lack of sleep, such as poor concentration, irritability and, of course, tiredness, some women choose to continue HRT purely for control of that symptom, even if they are not having flushes.

Some women find herbal drinks such as chamomile helpful, or sedative herbs such as valerian.

Joint aches

Joint aches commonly occur, often affecting neck, wrists and shoulders, but since other causes such as osteoarthritis are very common at this age, they may not be recognised as being associated with the menopause.

I started HRT because of hot flushes, which helped, but I was very surprised when my aching joints also got better. Could my aches and pains have been due to the menopause or was it just coincidence?

Joint aches are an often unrecognised but quite common symptom of the menopause. As well as the possible effect of lack of oestrogen affecting the ligaments around joints, research has also shown that this hormonal lack is involved in the development of osteoarthritis. Limited research has been shown that osteoarthritis is more common after the menopause and that use of oestrogen after the menopause may reduce the numbers of women developing the disease.

Weight gain

Do you think going through the menopause means I shall put on weight? I seem to have put on a stone since the menopause. I'm not eating any differently and I exercise as much as I ever have. My clothes feel tight and it makes me feel old and frumpy. Why does this happen?

Many women put on weight around the time of the menopause. When your hormone levels change at the menopause, it is thought that the rate at which you burn off calories (your metabolic rate) reduces. More fat is being stored than before, and so many women do both put on weight and change their shape. Fat is often redistributed and tends to increase around the waist, leading to the perception of weight gain, even if in some women the weight may not change much – 'bums to tums'! There is no magic, easy answer! Weight loss requires a combination of changing eating patterns and increasing exercise. This is often a time for a 'wake-up call' when diet and lifestyle need to be reviewed. We talk more about this in Chapter 7.

Breast tenderness

Over the last few months my breasts have been so sore, I can't bear them to be touched. I'm also having totally irregular and heavy periods. Are these connected and is it hormonal?

Breast tenderness is often a symptom of oestrogen excess and, although many of the menopausal and perimenopausal symptoms are due to oestrogen deficiency, symptoms of oestrogen excess can occur as the oestrogen levels are fluctuating. These fluctuating levels may also cause a change in periods. Fluid retention can also cause breast tenderness and is often associated with weight gain, correction of which can help. Evening primrose oil and starflower oil have been shown to reduce breast tenderness and wearing a good supportive bra is essential.

Psychological symptoms

Psychological symptoms such as mood swings, irritability, anxiety, difficulty concentrating, difficulty coping and forgetfulness may be related to hormonal changes, either directly or indirectly, e.g. due to sleep disturbance. However, other life events such as worry over elderly relatives, teenage children, and pressures from work commonly occur around the time of menopause and may contribute to such 'symptoms'.

My mum is going through 'the change' at the moment and she's often really bad tempered. She wasn't always like this. I find it difficult as I am the oldest, so I seem to get most of the flack! Is there anything I could suggest she does to make her feel better?

Being aware that mood changes often occur at this stage and being patient and understanding will be a huge help for your mum. Although you might feel that the brunt of the bad temper falls on you, trying very hard not to fight back is really important. At a 'calmer moment', sitting down with your mum and explaining that you understand will help her feel that she is not alone. Asking for ways in which the family can help will let her know that she has support through this difficult time. Many women cope for years with working and running the household with little time for themselves; with the onset of menopausal symptoms, this busy life becomes unsustainable, and help with even small tasks can be much appreciated. Suggesting that she speak to her doctor about possible treatment, or get more information from websites or books may also help.

Sexual problems

Sexual problems can be caused by vaginal dryness from low oestrogen levels, resulting in discomfort during intercourse. Effective treatments are available. As both men and women get older, interest in sex may decrease but this particularly affects women. Treatment of other menopausal symptoms may indirectly improve sexual desire (*libido*) by improving feelings of wellbeing and energy levels, e.g. by improving sleep through control of night sweats; however, restoring hormone levels can also improve sensation. Relationship problems have an obvious effect on libido, so hormonal treatment may not always be the 'magic' solution! Read more about this in Chapter 12.

HOW LONG DO SYMPTOMS LAST?

The duration of 'early' symptoms is very variable from a few months to many years and the severity varies between individuals. On average, 'early' symptoms last between 2 and 5 years.

My friend sailed through the menopause without any flushes but I'm still having them after 6 years. Am I doing something wrong?

Although the flush is the classic menopausal symptom that we've known about for many years, there is still much uncertainty about why they happen and the role of other non-hormonal factors. There are probably many other chemicals and hormones that interact to control how our internal thermostat works, and the balance will be different in every woman. The persistence of symptoms does not mean that it is your fault, but often diet and lifestyle factors can be adjusted to help.

My periods stopped 7 years ago. I did have some flushes then but only for a few months. Why have they come back now?

When flushes return after a gap, it is worth having blood tests to check for thyroid function and sugar level, since disorders of the thyroid gland and poor sugar control can cause similar symptoms to those of the menopause, and correction of these problems can treat the flushes. Menopausal flushes returning after a gap is unusual but possible and, if troublesome, the same treatment options used at an earlier stage can be considered.

LATER SYMPTOMS IN THE MENOPAUSE

Some later symptoms are due to the effects of oestrogen deficiency on the bladder and vagina and include:

- passing urine more often by day and/or by night
- discomfort on passing urine
- urine infection
- leakage of urine
- vaginal dryness, discomfort, burning and itching
- vaginal discharge
- discomfort during intercourse.

Other possible symptoms may also include:

- skin problems
- hair thinning or extra hair
- memory loss
- depression.

I have had lots of courses of antibiotics for cystitis but I've now been given some oestrogen pessaries – how can these help?

Often oestrogen deficiency causes cystitis-like symptoms, which don't respond to antibiotics. Oestrogen receptors are present in the base of the bladder, bladder muscle and the sphincter at the bladder opening so that, at the menopause, with less oestrogen around, these tissues very commonly weaken or become thin (*atrophy*). Symptoms may mimic cystitis and are often treated inappropriately with antibiotics. For bladder and vaginal symptoms, local vaginal oestrogen (tablets, cream, pessaries or ring) can be very helpful. Low dose, vaginal oestrogen can be used when systemic oestrogen (such as tablets or patches) is inappropriate, and can be continued in the long term with minimal risk of adverse effects. We talk more about this in Chapter 8.

> *Since the menopause, I've noticed a horrible discharge from my vagina. I feel dirty and embarrassed. I haven't done anything differently recently or changed my soap, so why is it happening?*

With the lack of oestrogen the acidity of the vagina changes allowing bacteria that aren't usually present to thrive. A course of antibiotics often helps but, to prevent the problem recurring, vaginal oestrogen can restore the correct acidity, allowing the correct balance of bacteria to be restored. Again, this is discussed more fully in Chapter 8.

> *I don't have very good bladder control anymore. Often, if I cough or sneeze, or don't get to the loo in time, I leak – it is so embarrassing. I have to wear pads, when I thought I wouldn't need to buy pads any more after my periods stopped! Can anything help?*

Loss of bladder control is a very common problem, yet is hugely underreported and undertreated, often because of embarrassment. Treatments include physiotherapy with specific exercises to improve the tone of your pelvic floor, retraining of your bladder, vaginal oestrogen and drugs, which can reduce bladder activity or improve the strength of your bladder support muscles. Chapter 7 discusses exercises that can help you, but see your doctor for a full assessment to plan the best treatment for you.

*My husband and I can't have sex anymore – it's too painful. I
know we're getting older but I don't think we are too old yet!
Although he's very understanding, I feel so bad about it and
want be able to enjoy sex again. What should we do?*

As with the bladder problems, this is also a very common problem
and effective treatments are available. The discomfort is often
due to the vaginal tissues becoming dry, thin and fragile because of
the lack of oestrogen. This can be helped by vaginal moisturisers,
lubricating gel or vaginal oestrogen in the form of a small tablet, pessary, cream or ring. Even if you don't want to, or have been advised
not to take HRT, vaginal oestrogen can often be used since the hormone is concentrated into the vagina and is unlikely to get into your
system. This is discussed further in Chapter 8.

*I've noticed that my hair is becoming thinner and I don't need
to cut my nails as often – is this menopause related?*

Other later menopausal symptoms include effects from changes in
collagen production, a protein found in skin, hair, nails and ten-
dons. Hair thinning, dryness and the growth of unwanted hair can
be explained by the lack of oestrogen and the relative excess of
androgens (male type hormones) in the menopause (the ovaries continue to produce some androgens, including testosterone, after the
menopause – their effect is no longer overridden by oestrogen).
However, hair loss may be more related to age rather than hormone
related, and response to HRT in this situation is unclear. Iron deficiency and thyroid disease can also cause hair loss and your doctor
may feel it is appropriate to test the levels of iron and thyroid hormone, particularly if there are other signs of these. Hair loss can also
be caused by stress.

My pubic hair has become so thin since the menopause. I feel old and less feminine. Why has this happened?

The fall in hormone levels, which occurs at the menopause and is also age related, can cause both head and pubic hair thinning. Unfortunately, very little information is available about the effects of oestrogen and testosterone levels on pubic hair changes, nor on the effects of treatment. Changes such as these are a sign of the body changing, but should not herald old age! If you think you are less feminine because of it, discuss your concerns with your partner and be reassured that your relationship need not be affected by this change.

Will I grow a beard when I become menopausal?

An increase in facial hair can occur as the hormone balance changes with a relative excess of androgens, but this is also an age-related feature. Most women have very few problems with hair growth so it is by no means an inevitable consequence of the menopause!

Will HRT rebalance the hormones and prevent facial hair?

Little, if any, research has examined the effect of HRT and facial hair. If this is a particular problem, it would seem logical to discuss with your doctor the possibility of using a type of HRT in which the progestogen part has minimal male hormone effect; there are different types of progestogens available as part of HRT preparations – some are related to androgens but others less so. If you have had the womb removed (hysterectomy), then usually progestogen is not required, so this would not be an issue and the oestrogen-only HRT may help.

My skin seems quite dry and I've developed wrinkles. Is it the menopause or is it just the fact that I'm getting older?

Collagen production (see an earlier question) is affected by falling oestrogen levels: the skin may become drier, thinner, less elastic, more prone to bruising and skin itching can occur. Occasionally, a 'crawling' sensation might be experienced, but it is unclear whether this is due to skin changes or changes in the peripheral nerves. Age and environmental factors also can cause problems.

It has been calculated that approximately 30% of skin collagen is lost during the first 5 years after the menopause, and then the decline slows to 2% per year after that. For many years it has been claimed that one of the benefits of HRT is to delay the effects of ageing on skin and many women have noticed an improvement in skin appearance and texture when taking HRT. This is discussed further in Chapter 8.

Other helpful measures include drinking plenty of water to keep the skin hydrated, not smoking, using a moisturising cream regularly and avoiding too much sun exposure; as we age, our skin is more susceptible to harmful rays, and we should use a sunscreen of factor 15 or more if we are exposed to the sun for more than 20 minutes.

I had lots of acne when I was a teenager. I can't believe it but the spots seem to be coming back with my menopause. I wouldn't mind if I also had the energy I had when I was a teenager! What on earth is going on?

Women can suffer from adult acne at the menopause because of the change in ratio of hormones: as oestrogen levels decrease, we still produce some testosterone and the balance changes, allowing testosterone to have an effect such as causing facial spots in a few women. It does not seem to be a common problem, nor to be long lasting.

Does the menopause cause memory loss? I am having terrible problems – I have to write numerous lists to help me. I can even forget what I was going to say in the middle of a sentence – it's awful!

Difficulty with concentration and memory loss have often been linked with the menopause, but is not clear whether there is a direct association with the hormone changes or whether the problems are due to a 'knock-on' effect from difficulty in sleeping, or, again, whether age-related changes are more important. Several studies that have looked at the effect of HRT on concentration and memory have often given inconclusive results, although many women do report an improvement. It is not clear if beneficial effects are a direct result of treatment with HRT or as a result of its improvement of symptoms such as night sweats and sleep patterns. Using simple aids such as lists can be very helpful and many people rely on such help increasingly.

I've just been diagnosed with depression and been prescribed some tablets. I haven't started them yet because I wonder if it's really the menopause that's causing it.

Although depressive moods and anxiety may be symptoms of the menopause, depressive illness is not necessarily caused by the menopause and can happen at any time. If you have been found to have clinical depression, then it should be treated as discussed with your doctor, but if the problems are more likely to be mood changes, especially if associated with other menopausal symptoms, then specific menopause treatment may be more appropriate. If you are worried about taking antidepressants, why not go back to your doctor and discuss it again?

4 | **Osteoporosis** by Katrina Martin

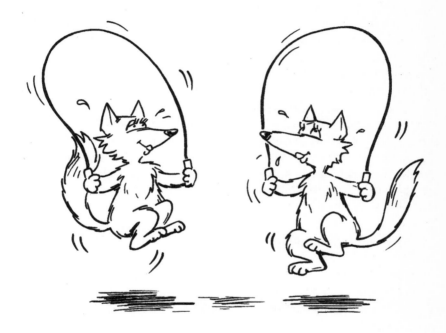

The most important long-term effect of the menopause is that of falling oestrogen levels on the bones. With age and reduced oestrogen levels, particularly when the menopause occurs before the age of 45, there is an increased risk of loss of bone strength causing bones to become thinner and more fragile (*osteoporosis*).

Osteoporosis is a progressive disease now estimated to affect one in two women over the age of 50. It is more common in women than in men because women have smaller, less dense bones, and because accelerated bone loss is experienced at the time of the menopause. It can be a major cause of pain and disability, but is preventable and treatable and is not always an inevitable consequence of the menopause.

WHAT IS OSTEOPOROSIS?

Osteoporosis literally means 'porous bones', although it is also defined as 'a systemic skeletal disease, characterised by low bone mass and micro-architectural deterioration of bone tissue, with a consequent increase in bone fragility and susceptibility to fracture'.

The bones in our skeleton are made up of a thick outer shell and a strong inner mesh; this looks like a honeycomb and consists of protein, calcium and other minerals. The honeycomb structure is made up of struts of bone with blood vessels and bone marrow in the spaces between (Fig. 4.1a). In osteoporosis, the struts of bone become thin and break, making the bones even more porous and fragile (Fig. 4.1b). This increased fragility can lead to bones breaking more easily even after a simple fall or bump, known as a 'low trauma fracture'. Often it is a fracture giving a warning sign that someone may have osteoporosis.

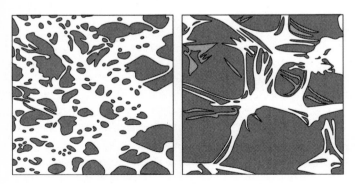

Figure 4.1 Healthy bone (**a**) and osteoporotic bone (**b**).

Bone formation

To understand more about osteoporosis and the effects of the menopause on bone strength, it is first important to understand the normal process of bone formation.

Bone is a highly specialised, living tissue, which is constantly changing and being renewed. Old bone is renewed by a process known as *bone remodelling*, or bone 'turnover'. This process basically involves cells called *osteoclasts* breaking down and removing old bone, and replacing it with new bone formed by cells called *osteoblasts*. The osteoblast cells fill the cavity created by removal of old bone, with new bone.

Does this process of bone formation continue throughout life?

Yes it does, but at a slower rate as you get older. In childhood and adolescence, the bone building cells (osteoblasts) work faster causing bones to increase in density and strength. Bones grow

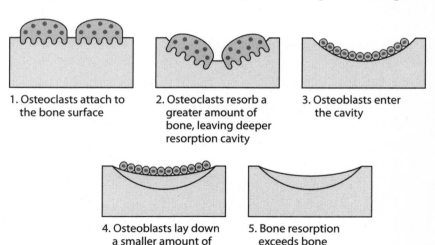

1. Osteoclasts attach to the bone surface

2. Osteoclasts resorb a greater amount of bone, leaving deeper resorption cavity

3. Osteoblasts enter the cavity

4. Osteoblasts lay down a smaller amount of bone than is resorbed

5. Bone resorption exceeds bone formation

Figure 4.2 Role of osteoclasts and osteoblasts in osteoporosis.

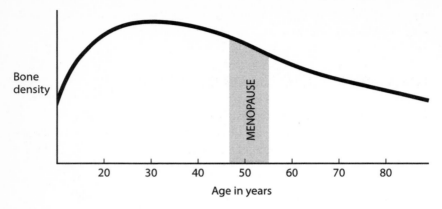

Figure 4.3 Decline in bone density with age.

rapidly and the whole skeleton can be renewed in 2 years, whereas in adulthood it takes 7–10 years as the bone remodelling process slows down. Bones continue to grow in strength until your mid- to late twenties when you reach your peak bone mass, i.e. when your bones have reached their maximum strength. Up until your mid- to late thirties, a balance between the activity of the osteoclasts and osteoblasts means that bone density levels out and is maintained. It then starts to decrease as part of the natural ageing process. See Figs 4.2 and 4.3.

What happens to my bones when I reach the menopause?

The age of the menopause is crucial to the rate of bone loss. At the menopause, which is usually around the age of 51, the ovaries produce lower levels of the hormone oestrogen, which is known to protect the bones by maintaining bone density and reducing fracture risk. The decrease in hormone levels accelerates bone loss, with most women experiencing about 1% of bone loss per year, although in some women this may be greater. At the age of 50, it is estimated that one-third of a woman's life will be spent without the bone-protective effects of oestrogen; therefore for younger menopausal women (below age 45), this length of time will be longer and their risk of osteoporosis greater.

OTHER RISK FACTORS FOR OSTEOPOROSIS

Reaching the menopause is only one factor that can increase your risk of osteoporosis. Most of our bone strength (70–80%) is genetically determined, but other factors include:

- breaking a bone after a minor fall (low trauma fracture)
- a family history of diagnosed osteoporosis
- your mother having a hip fracture
- long-term use of or high-dose oral steroid therapy
- medical conditions that may affect absorption of food, such as ulcerative colitis, Crohn's disease, coeliac disease, gastric surgery, or liver disease (see Chapter 11)
- amenorrhoea (absence of periods) for greater than 6 months, for reasons other than pregnancy (for example, eating disorders and excessive exercise), which reduces lifetime exposure to oestrogen
- smoking
- excess alcohol intake (more than 14 units per week where 1 unit = 1 measure of spirit or ½ pint of beer/lager or small 125 ml glass of wine)
- a diet low in calcium (less than 700 mg daily)
- lack of weight-bearing exercise, e.g. walking, jogging, running, aerobics
- being underweight
- other medical conditions, e.g. overactive thyroid, rheumatoid arthritis.

I broke my wrist after tripping and putting out my hand to save myself when I fell. Does this mean I have osteoporosis?

No, not necessarily, but this can be a warning sign that your bones are thinner and more fragile than normal, and it is worth being investigated. As osteoporosis is known as the ' silent disease', in that it does not cause any symptoms, often a simple fracture can be the first sign. Fractures of the wrist, spine and hip are the most common and can cause considerable pain, disability and sometimes death.

Other signs can be loss of height and curvature of the spine (*kyphosis*), commonly known as a 'dowager's hump'.

My mother had a hip fracture and was found to have osteoporosis. I am worried that the same will happen to me, especially when I become menopausal. What can I do?

As most of our bone strength is genetically determined, your mother's history can increase your risk of osteoporosis. Fractures of the wrist, spine and hip are commonly associated with osteoporosis, and nowadays there are some very effective treatments available for treating osteoporosis and reducing the risk of further fractures (see later section in this chapter). It may well be that your mother had other risk factors, such as an early menopause, which contributed to her osteoporosis and subsequent fracture. As well as dietary and lifestyle measures (see below), you may want to consider starting HRT when you reach the menopause, as this is useful for women who have menopausal symptoms and risk factors for osteoporosis – recent studies have confirmed that it can help to reduce the risk of fractures. Measures such as a healthy, calcium-rich diet and regular weight-bearing exercise, as well as keeping your own risk factors to a minimum by not smoking and not drinking too much alcohol for example, can also help. A DEXA scan (see below), may also be advisable, particularly if it will influence your decision on whether or not to start treatment, such as HRT, at the time of your own menopause.

I am 55 years old, have been on HRT for 5 years but recently came off it. I have no flushes and feel fine. I am, however, concerned that I will now develop osteoporosis as my mother had osteoporosis and a severe curvature of the spine. What should I do?

First of all, it is important to keep your own risk factors to a minimum by having a healthy, varied diet with lots of calcium-rich foods, taking regular weight-bearing exercise, not smoking and not having excessive amounts of alcohol (see later section in this chapter). While you have been on HRT this should have given you some bone protection; however, it is likely that your bone density will reduce a little now that you have stopped HRT, particularly in the next 1–2 years. It is difficult to know who loses bone strength at a faster rate than others: therefore it may be worthwhile having a DEXA scan (see below) in the next year or two to assess your bone density, particularly in view of your mother's history. The results of this scan can then help your doctor decide whether any further treatment for your bones is required. It is worth mentioning, however, that the risk of a woman of your age breaking a bone, even if you have osteoporosis, is very small, and this should be kept in mind when you discuss with your doctor whether any further treatment is required.

I have been on steroid tablets now for 3 months for polymyalgia rheumatica. Initally I was on a high dose and, although I am now on a lower dose, it is likely that I will be on steroids for some time, as each time my doctor tries to stop them my symptoms flare up. He has now prescribed me a weekly bisphosphonate tablet to protect my bones. Why is this and how long do I need to take it?

Glucocorticoids (steroids) are drugs used to reduce inflammation in many medical conditions such as polymyalgia, rheumatoid arthritis, asthma and inflammatory bowel disease. The most commonly prescribed oral steroid is prednisolone, and these drugs are usually used only when really needed, for example in an acute flare up of asthma where inhaled steroids alone may not be enough to manage the condition.

Steroids can be very helpful in managing certain medical conditions, and indeed seem to have helped you, but the down side is that they can increase the risk of osteoporosis and fracture, particularly when used on a long-term basis (for 3 months or more), or when required in frequent high doses. Any dose of steroid taken for more than 3 months can increase risk, although the greatest risk would seem to be associated with higher doses. Loss of bone density is greatest in the first 6 months of steroid treatment but fracture risk declines rapidly on stopping treatment. This is why your own doctor has now recommended that you take the bisphosphonate medication to protect your bones, as it seems that you will need steroids in the longer term. It is likely that you will continue on the bisphosphonate treatment as long as you are on your steroids. (There is a question on bisphosphonates later in this chapter.) Your doctor will advise you when and how to stop your steroids. Current recommendations are that those people at high risk of osteoporosis, for example those aged 65 and over, and those who have had a low trauma fracture, should start treatment to protect their bones when they start their steroid therapy, if it is likely that they will be on steroids for 3 months or more. For those under age 65, who have not had a low trauma fracture, or have other risk factors for osteoporosis, then a DEXA scan is recommended to assess the need for appropriate bone-protective treatment.

It is also important, of course, in order to reduce your overall risk of osteoporosis, to have a good, healthy, calcium-rich diet, take regular weight-bearing exercise, not smoke and keep alcohol to moderation (see later section).

I am on a steroid inhaler for asthma. Does this have the same effect on bones as the tablets?

Steroids taken in an inhaled form usually involve smaller doses than taking oral steroids and therefore the effects on bone density and fracture risk may be less. Effects are less certain, however, and some studies have shown an increase in bone loss with higher dose treatments. Lots of people need to use steroid inhalers to control their asthma and, if they are taken in this way, often the need for oral steroids, where the osteoporosis and fracture risk is greater, is avoided. However, if you are using a high dose of inhaled steroid and have other risk factors for osteoporosis, then a DEXA scan may be required to assess your need for appropriate bone-protective treatment. Again, following dietary and lifestyle advice for bone health is important.

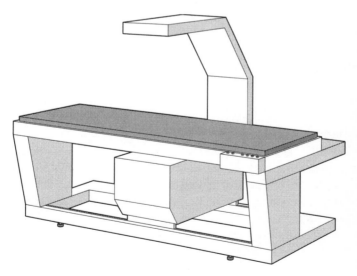

Figure 4.4 DEXA scanning machine.

TESTS FOR OSTEOPOROSIS

The most accurate test currently available for determining whether you have osteoporosis is called a *dual energy X-ray absorptiometry (DEXA)* scan (a bone *densitometry* test). This is a simple type of radiograph, which involves using low doses of radiation (less than used for a chest radiograph) to measure bone density. It involves you lying on a firm couch whilst an X-ray arm passes over you. It does not involve you going into a 'tunnel' and is a painless procedure taking about 10 minutes. Bone density measurements are usually taken of the lower spine and hips. This gives an overall prediction of your bone mineral density and can help to predict your risk of breaking a bone. It is usually used to diagnose osteoporosis in those people who are at highest risk. Access to DEXA scanning services varies, however, so it would be worthwhile you checking with your doctor to see if it is available in your area.

I have been taking HRT for control of flushes and sweats since my early menopause. Should I have a DEXA scan to check my bones?

No not necessarily, as it is likely that the HRT is protecting your bones while you are taking it. Even most low-dose preparations are now licensed for bone protection but, if in doubt, check with your doctor. Other risk factors also need to be taken into account and your individual risk for osteoporosis assessed. Most women who have an early menopause can continue taking HRT up until the age of 50, the average age of the menopause, by which time the risk of osteoporosis associated with an early menopause will be lessened. If you then stop HRT and no longer require it for symptom control, but have other risk factors for osteoporosis, then a DEXA scan may be worthwhile at that stage to determine whether any other treatment is required.

My doctor has told me that my DEXA scan showed osteopenia.
What does this mean?

Osteopenia means that there has been some bone thinning but not enough to be diagnosed as osteoporosis. It means that your bones are not dense enough to be in the normal range but not thin enough to be in the osteoporosis category. They are somewhere in between. Being in the osteopenia category does not always mean that treatment is required for your bones, as this level of bone density may be what is expected for someone of your age, and does not necessarily mean that you are at an increased risk of breaking a bone. Treatment depends on factors such as age, degree of osteopenia, and other risk factors for osteoporosis including whether you have broken any bones. Dietary and lifestyle measures are also important (see Chapter 7).

I have just had a DEXA scan and found that I have
osteoporosis, which surprised me as I did not go through the
menopause until my mid-50s, have always had a good
healthy diet, been fit and active and have never smoked. My
daughters, who are in their 30s, are now worried that they
might develop it, and wondered whether they should have a
DEXA scan too?

Although there are lots of reasons why we can develop osteoporosis, sometimes the actual cause is unknown. This is known as *idiopathic osteoporosis*. Also, our risk of osteoporosis is largely hereditary, so it may well be that genetic factors are the main reason why you have osteoporosis. It can be frustrating to think that you have kept your own risk factors for osteoporosis low and still have the disease; however, dietary and lifestyle factors are still important in preventing and managing osteoporosis and this is the main advice that your daughters should follow. As they are young women, they are likely to still be having periods and therefore have the protection of oestrogen on their bones, so at this stage a DEXA scan is probably not worthwhile. It may, however, be worth considering when they reach their menopause, as bone density does decrease more quickly at this time. In the meantime, the usual dietary and lifestyle advice of not smoking, not overindulging in alcohol, having a varied, healthy diet with plenty of foods rich in calcium, and taking regular weight-bearing exercise remains important.

TREATMENT

Hormone replacement protection

Is it true that taking HRT will protect my bones?

Although, for many women, the main reason for taking HRT is for control of menopausal symptoms, it has been shown to maintain bone density while being taken, and to help reduce the risk of breaking a bone. Although it is not used as a first-line treatment for osteoporosis, HRT is particularly useful in the prevention of osteoporosis in those women who have an early menopause, as well as for those who require it to help menopausal symptoms. It is very effective at preventing bone loss and can be used if other treatments (see next section) are not suitable or are difficult to take.

How long should I take HRT to protect my bones?

The length of time HRT is taken for bone protection depends on a number of factors including age of menopause, age of starting HRT, family history of osteoporosis and other risk factors. The risks and benefits of HRT need to be assessed on an individual basis, and the use of HRT should be reviewed and discussed on a yearly basis. If you have started HRT for an early menopause, then it can be taken until you are 50, the average age of the menopause, when the risks and benefits of continuing HRT should then be discussed and evaluated further with your doctor or practice nurse.

I had breast cancer and cannot take HRT, so what can I do to keep my bones strong?

HRT is not suitable or indeed necessary for all women. Some women do not need HRT for symptom control, have medical reasons that contraindicate its use, or merely prefer not to take it. Although it is known that HRT offers bone protection, dietary and lifestyle measures are also important for bone health and, although important at all stages of life, are particularly important at the time of the menopause when bone loss is accelerated. Such measures include having a healthy varied diet with plenty of foods rich in calcium, not having too much caffeine, not overindulging in alcohol, not smoking, and taking regular weight-bearing exercise such as walking.

There are other non-hormonal drugs available (see later section in this chapter) for the prevention and treatment of osteoporosis; however, the suitability of these drugs is determined by such factors as your age, whether you have previously broken a bone, any other risk factors, and whether you have actual osteoporosis or not. Like HRT, the risks and benefits of these treatments have to be considered on an individual basis.

Other drug therapies

My mother has been prescribed a tablet for her bones, which she has to take on an empty stomach once a week. Why is this and what does this drug do?

Your mum will be taking one of the bisphosphonate drugs. These drugs are non-hormonal and work by affecting bone resorption. Basically this means that they slow down the action of the cells that break down bone (osteoclasts), allowing the bone-building cells (osteoblasts) to work more effectively in laying down new bone and increasing bone density. We have discussed how bone is formed earlier in this chapter. The bisphosphonate drugs have been shown to be very effective in increasing bone strength and reducing fracture risk. There are currently four bisphosphonates available to treat osteo-porosis: etidronate (Didronel), alendronate (Fosamax), risedronate (Actonel) and, the newest, ibandronate (Bonviva). Your mother will be on either alendronate or risedronate, which are available as weekly tablets, as well as in daily form. These types of drugs are not well absorbed from the gut and can cause some stomach problems, such as indigestion and heartburn in some people, although gener-ally they are very well tolerated. To maximise absorption and reduce the risk of stomach upset, these drugs have to be taken on an empty stomach with a glass of plain tap water, at least ½ hour before any other fluids, food or medications. It is also advised that you do not lie flat after taking these drugs, to allow the tablet to stay in the stomach and be absorbed. As this advice has to be followed in detail for these drugs to work effectively, most people prefer the weekly to the daily regime. The newest of the bisphosphonate drugs, ibandronate, com-monly known as Bonviva, is available as a monthly tablet.

Now that I am postmenopausal, I worry both about my bones and joints. I am taking alendronate for my bones, but what do you think about chondroitin/glucosamine for joints?

Glucosamine is a naturally occurring sugar that is used in the formation of components of joint cartilage. It can be found in some foods such as shellfish and is available in supplement form. Glucosamine is often used for pain relief in osteoarthritis and other joint disorders. Several trials have demonstrated a moderate benefi-cial effect on pain relief and a recent review concluded that glucosamine 1500 mg daily is a reasonable choice for treatment of osteoarthritis of the knee, but further information is required on its effect at other sites. It may take up to 1 month for benefits to be apparent. Side effects appear to be mild and infrequent, and include nausea, vomiting, constipation, diarrhoea, dyspepsia, rash, drowsi-ness, headache and insomnia. There are no known drug interactions between glucosamine and other medicines. It should be used with caution if you are allergic to shellfish since some glucosamine products may be derived from shellfish sources.

I have read about a new injection for osteoporosis. As I have not been able to take the bisphosphonate drugs because of ongoing stomach problems, I wondered if I could have this new injection to treat my osteoporosis?

The injection you have read about is parathyroid hormone, or teriparatide. It is commonly known as Forsteo and it works in a different way to other osteoporosis drugs: it stimulates the bone-building cells to form new bone rather than reducing the resorption of bone cells. It is available as a daily injection in an insulin-type pen, which you are taught to give yourself. It is currently available as an 18-month treatment, and is only prescribed by specialist osteoporosis centres. It is usually used in postmenopausal women who have severe osteoporosis and fractures. Prescription of this drug would therefore depend on several factors including the severity of osteoporosis, your fracture history and response to other treatments.

I have been reading about another drug called Protelos. Would I be able to have this?

This is another new treatment. Its generic name is strontium ranelate (the chemical name) and its brand name is Protelos (the drug company's name for it). It comes in a 2 g sachet and is taken daily at bedtime. It is the first osteoporosis drug that works by both slowing down the action of the cells that break down bone as well as stimulating the bone-building cells to build new bone – it is therefore known as a dual action bone agent (DABA). It is taken in a glass of water each night at least 2 hours after eating and is well tolerated. Any calcium supplements should be taken at least 2 hours before to allow the drug to be absorbed properly. It has been shown to reduce the risk of hip and spinal (vertebral) fractures. You would be prescribed this only if you cannot tolerate the bisphosphonate drugs.

My doctor has mentioned a drug called raloxifene as a possible
treatment for osteoporosis, which I have in my spine. He called
it a SERM – what does this mean?

Raloxifene (commonly known as Evista) is a drug known as a selective oestrogen receptor modulator or SERM for short. It works by binding only to some oestrogen receptors in the body and, by doing so, works in a similar way to oestrogen on bones, but not so in tissues like the breast where it has an antioestrogen effect. It therefore has a protective effect on bones without increasing the risk of breast cancer, which is associated with the long-term use of HRT in women over the age of 50. It is in fact thought to reduce the risk of breast cancer. It also does not stimulate the lining of the womb, so any menstrual bleeding or spotting is avoided. It is used for the prevention and treatment of osteoporosis in postmenopausal women and has been shown to reduce the risk of fractures of the spine.

It is taken as a daily tablet in a dose of 60 mg. Like HRT, it does cause a small increased risk of blood clots, such as deep vein thrombosis (DVT) and can sometimes cause or worsen flushes. It is therefore most suitable for women who are not having such menopausal symptoms.

Diet and lifestyle

We discuss these aspects more fully in Chapter 7, but we answer some questions here that relate specifically to osteoporosis.

I think I eat a healthy and varied diet. Should I be following
a special type of diet to keep my bones strong?

Generally a healthy, well-balanced diet with foods from the four main food groups is all that is required:

- Aim for five portions of fruit or vegetables per day to ensure adequate vitamins and minerals.

- Include carbohydrates, such as bread, potatoes, pasta and cereals.

- Add proteins, such as meat, eggs, fish and pulses.

- Finally eat plenty of calcium-rich foods, such as milk, cheese, and other dairy products.

All these should provide a varied diet with the necessary nutrients for healthy bones. Bones particularly need calcium and, as we get older, we tend to absorb less calcium, which means that extra efforts may be required to ensure an adequate calcium intake. Dairy products are the easiest and richest sources of calcium: a pint of semi-skimmed milk equals your recommended daily requirement of 700 mg. However, non-dairy foods such as green, leafy vegetables, bread, cereals and baked beans also contain calcium, although you would probably need to eat more of these types of foods to ensure that you are getting enough. People who have osteoporosis may need more calcium and should aim for about 1200 mg per day.

I have high cholesterol and have been avoiding dairy products. What should I do to make sure that I get enough calcium?

Actually, low-fat dairy products, such as skimmed and semi-skimmed milk, low-fat cheeses and yoghurts, contain a little more calcium than full-cream products, as calcium is mainly in the non-cream part of milk. It seems to be a common misconception that you have to have full cream products to get the most calcium but actually you can reap the benefits without the fat!

I have heard that vitamin D is important for strong bones. Is this so, and how can I make sure that I get enough?

Yes, vitamin D is important as it helps calcium to be absorbed properly from the gut. Foods such as dairy products, eggs, oily fish and fortified margarines are good sources of vitamin D, but most of our supply is obtained from the action of sunlight on the skin. It is estimated that about 50% of people with osteoporosis are deficient in vitamin D, and deficiency is more common in the elderly and house-bound who may have little exposure to sunlight, who may have a poor dietary intake and who are less able to make their own supply. In such cases a calcium and vitamin D supplement may be worth-while to ensure adequate levels.

I enjoy swimming and go two to three times a week. Is this good for my bones?

Swimming is a good form of exercise for overall fitness and can help to keep joints flexible. It is not, however, a 'weight-bearing' exercise, as you do not support your weight through your bones when swimming. Walking about in the water or doing aquarobics, however, is more beneficial and can help with balance. Swimming and hydrotherapy can also be very relaxing on muscles and joints, and can help to relieve pain in people who may have had fractures because of osteoporosis.

I walk my dogs each day for half an hour. Is this enough to exercise my bones?

Any exercise is better than none. Walking is a good form of weight-bearing exercise. For a more beneficial effect, walk at a brisk pace over a distance. Walking helps to keep muscles as well as bones strong, helping to maintain balance and reducing the risk of falls. Other examples of weight-bearing exercise are:

- dancing
- jogging
- running
- tennis

- aerobics, and

- skipping.

Choose an activity that you enjoy and try and exercise at least two to three times a week. Short bursts of exercise such as going up and down stairs are also beneficial. Simple changes, such as walking more rather than taking the car, and climbing the stairs rather than taking the lift can make a difference.

I enjoy an occasional glass of wine, but a friend told me that alcohol is bad for your bones. Is this true?

Alcohol in moderation is fine; however, excessive amounts of alcohol can damage your bones. The recommended limit for women is 14 units per week with 1 unit being the equivalent of a small glass of wine, 1 measure of spirits or half a pint of pint of beer or cider. (Of course, home measures may be more, so be careful!)

Also, 'binge' drinking every so often can be just as harmful to bones as drinking on a regular basis, but a little of what you fancy should do no harm!

I know smoking is bad for your bones but I smoke only five to ten a day. Does that make a difference?

Ideally, if you are a smoker you should try and give up altogether, as smoking has a toxic effect on bone and can increase the risk of breaking a bone in later life. Smoking can also cause women to have an earlier menopause, which in turn can also affect bone strength, as well as sometimes worsening symptoms like flushes and sweats in women going through the menopause. Giving up smoking can only be good, with benefits not only to your bones, but to your heart, lungs and overall health and fitness.

5 | Menopause after hysterectomy

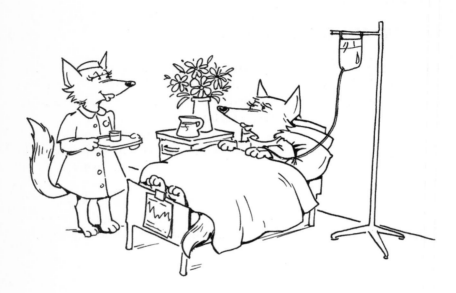

Many women undergo hysterectomy (surgical removal of the uterus or womb) for various gynaecological reasons. These include intolerable periods not controlled by medical means, fibroids, *endometriosis*, prolapse, and malignant or premalignant changes of the uterus, cervix or ovary.

Vaginal hysterectomy is when the uterus is removed through the top of the vagina and abdominal hysterectomy is when it is removed through the wall of the abdomen. Generally, recovery is quicker after a vaginal hysterectomy than after an abdominal procedure. The type chosen will depend on factors such as the reason for the operation and the surgeon's expertise.

If the ovaries are removed (oophorectomy) at the time of the hysterectomy, a sudden loss of ovarian hormone production, in particular oestrogen, occurs. This sudden, surgical menopause may cause oestrogen deficiency symptoms within a few days of the operation. These symptoms include hot flushes and sweats.

WHAT TYPE OF HYSTERECTOMY?

Hysterectomy can either be **total**, where both the uterus and cervix are removed, or **subtotal**, where the main part of the uterus is removed but the cervix is retained. If the cervix is retained, regular cervical screening by smears should be continued.

> *I had a hysterectomy 2 years ago and my doctor has asked me to go for a smear – I didn't think I needed cervical screening anymore.*

If the hysterectomy was a total hysterectomy, meaning removal of the neck of the uterus (cervix) as well as the main part of the

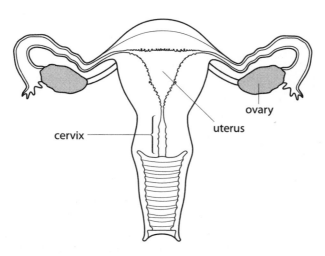

Figure 5.1 Position of uterus, cervix and ovaries.

uterus, then smears shouldn't be needed. If, however, the cervix was not removed at the time, then smears will need to be continued as before. It should be possible to find out from your doctor exactly which operation was carried out. Smears from the top of the vagina may also be recommended if cancerous changes were found in the cervix at the time of the hysterectomy.

I am about to have a hysterectomy on the advice of my doctor. The consultant has given me a choice of leaving my ovaries in. I'm not sure what to do.

At the time of a hysterectomy, the ovaries can be conserved (left behind) or removed. The decision as to which type of hysterectomy is needed will be determined by what type of gynaecological problem you have, by your past medical history, your age and by your family history. The final choice will be up to you.

If one or both ovaries are conserved at the time of hysterectomy, three scenarios are possible:

- **Continuing normal ovarian function.** The ovaries may continue producing hormones in their cyclical manner until the normal age of the menopause (usually 50 to 54 years of age, average age 51 years). This normal cyclical hormone production may cause symptoms of *premenstrual syndrome* (PMS), even in the absence of periods. This is because PMS symptoms are due to the changing hormone levels, and not due to the presence of bleeding. Oestrogen deficiency symptoms, if they occur, would happen at the normal menopausal age.

- **Early ovarian failure – apparent.** Following a hysterectomy, the ovaries may stop producing hormones sooner than expected. This can even happen within 1–2 years following the hysterectomy and is thought to be due to an interference with the blood supply to the ovaries at the time of the hysterectomy. Studies looking at the function of the ovaries following a hysterectomy have shown varying results about the possibility of subsequent ovarian failure, but do seem to show that the ovaries may fail at an earlier age than normal. When ovarian failure is apparent, menopausal symptoms will be noticed. If this happens, it is very important that these symptoms and the possible use of HRT are discussed with a doctor or practice nurse.

- **Early ovarian failure – silent**. In some women, the conserved ovaries may fail early but the falling oestrogen level may not cause the usual signs of oestrogen deficiency. Since there are no periods after a hysterectomy, the usual change in periods that follows a change in ovarian function is absent and so early menopause may go unnoticed. It therefore may be recommended that, following a hysterectomy with one or both ovaries conserved before the age of 45, a blood test should be taken approximately once a year to check hormone levels for evidence of an early menopause. If menopausal symptoms have developed, blood tests are not required.

It is important to report symptoms of early ovarian failure, or to detect silent early ovarian failure for the following reasons:

- Oestrogen deficiency symptoms can be unpleasant and effective therapy is available.

- Oestrogen is very good for maintaining bone strength. If your production of oestrogen is lost at an early age (before 45 years), then you may have an increased risk of osteoporosis (bone thinning). However, very effective treatments are now available to both prevent and treat osteoporosis (see Chapter 4). The early loss of oestrogen may also increase the risk of heart disease, but the use of HRT following early menopause is currently thought to protect the heart.

I've had a hysterectomy but kept my ovaries. What happens to my eggs and can I still get pregnant?

The ovaries, while continuing to function, will release an egg or two each month but these will be absorbed in the cavity of the abdomen and pregnancy is not possible as sperm cannot reach the eggs for fertilisation to occur.

I had a hysterectomy when I was 30. My ovaries were kept. I'm now 38 and having awful sweats. My friend told me that it can't be the menopause because I'm too young – what can be wrong?

Although other conditions such as thyroid problems can cause similar symptoms, it is possible that the sweats are due to ovarian failure. As mentioned in the question above, there is some evidence that, after a hysterectomy, even without the ovaries being removed, the ovaries can fail at an earlier age than in women who have not had a hysterectomy. What we don't know is when you would have become menopausal if you hadn't had the hysterectomy. Whether or not this is happening early because of your hysterectomy, it is important to seek help. Although you are younger than the average age for the menopause, you are certainly not too young to be having menopausal symptoms – your doctor can discuss with you what treatment is available.

What will happen to my body after a hysterectomy – won't there be a gaping hole?

During a hysterectomy, the uterus and cervix are separated from the top of the vagina and the vagina is then closed over with absorbable stitches. Therefore there will not be a hole at the top of the vagina. Some women wonder what happens to the area in the pelvis where the uterus was. This area is quite small and is occupied by the bowel without leaving a large gap.

I've been advised to have a hysterectomy because I have large fibroids. What exactly are fibroids and why have I got them?

Fibroids are a benign (non-malignant) tumour or swelling in the muscle layer of the womb. They are very common and can vary in number and size, sometimes becoming extremely large. Fibroids can cause problems with discomfort and period problems. There is no specific reason why some women develop fibroids.

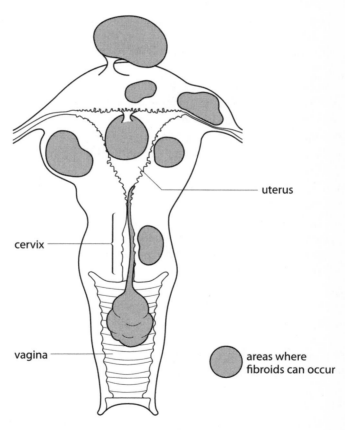

uterus

cervix

vagina

areas where fibroids can occur

Figure 5.2 Areas where fibroids can commonly occur.

How long will my menopausal symptoms go on for after I've had a hysterectomy?

As with menopausal symptoms after a natural menopause, there is no way of predicting how long your symptoms will continue for. The average duration of symptoms, such as hot flushes, is 2 years, but this might be longer or shorter. Undergoing a menopause because you've had a hysterectomy is not known to have any influence over duration of symptoms compared with a natural menopause.

I have been having difficult symptoms (heavy, irregular bleeding, hot flushes and mood swings) for 4 years now. My mother was the same for 8 years but then she had a hysterectomy and felt fine. I asked my doctor if I could have one, but he doesn't seem very keen. Why?

Over the last 10 years or so, other very effective treatments for period problems have been developed, which are much less invasive and safer than a hysterectomy. Doctors will now recommend that women with problem periods try simpler options first, such as medical treatment, the hormone-releasing coil containing levonorgestrel (such as Mirena), or endometrial ablation (treatment whereby the lining of the womb is destroyed without removing the womb). There is still a place for hysterectomies, but in many women they are not necessary. Further, if you are having hot flushes, you may well be in the perimenopause, and you should take into consideration that the menopause, with your periods stopping, might occur in the foreseeable future, although one can never predict when that may be. Simple treatments may therefore be all that is required to control bleeding until that time.

HYSTERECTOMY AND LOSS OF LIBIDO

I am going to have a hysterectomy in a few weeks' time. I've heard that some women feel less sexy after it. Will I feel less feminine do you think?

Some women view a hysterectomy as a loss of womanhood and femininity, though this is unusual. You should have a hysterectomy only after a full discussion and consideration of all options for your particular problem. Women sometimes regret having the operation if they feel that they were pushed into having the procedure without a full discussion. The ovarian hormones are responsible for 'femininity' and therefore keeping the ovaries, or taking hormone replacement after the hysterectomy if indicated, can maintain the hormone balance. For most women who have a hysterectomy for significant problems such as very heavy periods uncontrolled by other means, a hysterectomy can be a permanent cure and can hugely improve quality of life without regret.

Not long after my hysterectomy at the age of 49 (when both my ovaries were removed), I started to feel really unsexy. I couldn't be bothered to have sex with my husband and, of course, this is worrying him and myself. What can I do about it?

As well as causing a sudden drop in production of oestrogen, removal of the ovaries also causes a drop in testosterone production; in women, the ovaries are the main site of production of testosterone. After removal of both ovaries in premenopausal women, there is thought to be a drop of circulating testosterone levels of about 50%. Some health professionals therefore believe that after removal of ovaries, testosterone replacement should be offered along with oestrogen replacement, to counteract the effects of low testosterone, such as low libido, low mood and reduced energy levels. However, there is much debate about the role of testosterone and, if replacement is to be given, there is uncertainty about the best way for it to be taken by women and how it should be monitored. There is also concern about possible side effects. You should have a good discussion with a health professional about all the aspects before you make up your mind about what to do.

Will I still be able to have sex after my operation and will it be different?

Sexual activity can resume about 6 weeks after a hysterectomy by which time the tissues should be well healed. Some women have a hysterectomy because of problems that originally caused pain during intercourse. A hysterectomy in this situation can lead to less painful and more enjoyable sex. There is no reason why sexual enjoyment should be affected after a hysterectomy. If the ovaries have been removed as well, the fall in oestrogen levels may affect sexual activity due to consequent vaginal dryness and discomfort along with reduced interest. There is some evidence that removal of the ovaries can also affect sexual interest and response by reducing the ovarian source of testosterone. However, there are conflicting reports of the association between testosterone levels and sexual activity, and hence it is unclear whether or not women who have had removal of ovaries should be offered testosterone replacement along with oestrogen replacement.

HRT AND HYSTERECTOMY

If 'surgical menopause' (i.e. menopause occurring because both ovaries have been removed) occurs before the age of 45 years, the risk of osteoporosis is increased. HRT should then be considered for control of symptoms and/or for its protective effect on bone. You should decide whether or not to commence HRT after a full discussion with a health professional. This decision will be influenced by factors such as your age at the time of operation, past history (including any medical reasons why HRT should not be taken) and family history. HRT is usually recommended if the operation causes an early menopause because of the significantly increased risk of osteoporosis.

I started HRT after my hysterectomy when I was 41, 6 years ago. I'm wondering if I should stop it now since I've heard that you can take HRT only for 5 years.

The idea that HRT should be taken only for 5 years has come from the scientific evidence that there appears to be an increased risk of breast cancer if HRT is taken for more than 5 years. However, this finding applies to women who take HRT for more than 5 years after the normal age of menopause, in other words after the age of 50 years. For women who go into an early menopause for whatever reason, it is generally recommended that they can take HRT up to the age of 50 with minimal risk.

If HRT is commenced because of an early menopause after surgery, it can be continued until the age of 50 years without concern about the increased risk of breast cancer. The risk of breast cancer from HRT taken from the time of an early menopause up to the age of 50 is thought to be similar to the risk for someone who continues having a normal menstrual cycle up to the age of 50. However, it is thought that having an early surgical menopause and not taking HRT reduces the risk of breast cancer, but increases the risk of osteoporosis. Generally, following an early menopause for whatever reason, it is recommended that HRT is taken up to the age of 50 years. At around the age of 50, the decision as to whether or not to continue HRT should be made. This is the same decision that any woman becoming menopausal at the normal menopausal age would have to make, i.e. whether or not to commence HRT.

There is much more about HRT in Chapter 8.

I am due to have a hysterectomy and have my ovaries removed in a few months time. I am 43 and have had problems with my periods and cysts on my ovaries. What will happen to my hormones – do I go straight into the menopause and how will I know whether or not to take HRT?

If your ovaries are to be removed (oophorectomy) at the time of the hysterectomy, you will experience a sudden loss of ovarian hormone production, in particular oestrogen. This sudden, 'surgical menopause' may cause oestrogen deficiency symptoms within a few days of the operation. These symptoms include hot flushes and sweats. As you are under 45 years, the risk of osteoporosis is increased. You will be offered HRT for control of any symptoms and/or for its protective effect on bone. You should decide whether or not to start HRT after a full discussion with a health professional. This decision will be influenced by factors such as your age at the time of operation, past history (including any medical reasons why HRT should not be taken) and family history. HRT is usually recommended if the operation causes an early menopause (which is probably true in your case as you are under 45 years) because of the significant increased risk of osteoporosis.

There seem to be lots of different sorts of HRT preparations. What type do you recommend now that I have had a hysterectomy?

If HRT is started following a hysterectomy, it is usually prescribed as an oestrogen-only preparation; progestogen in addition is required only to protect the lining of the womb from becoming stimulated and thickened by the oestrogen. When the womb has been removed, there is no longer any lining present to become thickened, so oestrogen can be given on its own. This can be taken as a daily tablet, a weekly or twice weekly patch, a daily gel, a daily nasal spray, or a 6-monthly implant. The particular type of prescription is tailored to suit your own needs and will be offered by your doctor after consideration of your own preference, past history and, of course, cost. The most common prescription is oestrogen HRT as a daily tablet.

HRT using a combination of oestrogen and progestogen (which is recommended when the uterus is still present) is sometimes used after a hysterectomy if widespread endometriosis is found at the time of surgery – we discuss this in the next question.

I had a hysterectomy a couple of years ago. I've been on HRT (oestrogen only) but have now been told that I have endometriosis. What exactly is this and can anything be done?

Endometriosis is the presence of deposits of the lining of the uterus (*endometrium*) outside the uterus, e.g. on the ovaries, bladder, bowel and other organs in the body. These deposits are sensitive to the hormones produced by the ovaries. After hysterectomy and removal of the ovaries, there have been reports of deposits of endometriosis being stimulated following oestrogen-only HRT. It is thought that oestrogen combined with progestogen HRT is less likely to cause stimulation of these deposits, although there is little scientific evidence to support this – it will be a good idea to discuss the pros and cons about the possibility of taking a combined type of HRT.

After my hysterectomy and having my ovaries removed, I've been taking HRT. I don't suffer from hot flushes, in fact no problems like that at all, but I've no interest in sex and always feel tired. My doctor suggested trying some testosterone along with my HRT but I'm worried that I might develop male characteristics like developing a beard or a deep voice. Is that likely?

The problems that you are having may be due to the reduced levels of testosterone following removal of the ovaries. Although by no means do all women who have their ovaries removed require testosterone replacement, some do seem to benefit from it and a trial of testosterone would be worthwhile. At the moment there are very few ways in which testosterone is licensed for women. Your doctor may suggest a testosterone implant, which is a small pellet placed under the skin of the abdomen. Alternatively, a testosterone gel or patch, available at the moment for men, might be suggested for you but in a much smaller dose. Your blood levels would probably be measured to make sure you're not developing levels that are too high. If you are monitored regularly, then you are very unlikely to develop significant facial hair or a deep voice! Some increase in facial hair is quite common but reversible. Voice deepening is very rare but irreversible. If you find that testosterone helps, then it would be worth continuing. It may well be that other forms of testosterone replacement for women will become available in the future.

I am about to undergo a hysterectomy. I have asked the consultant if I could keep my cervix, as there have been lots of reports in the media about the possibility of loss of libido and not having 'good sex' without it. I'm not sure what to do about taking HRT.

The previous reports of improved sex life after a hysterectomy in which the cervix is retained (subtotal hysterectomy), compared with hysterectomy that includes removal of the cervix (total hysterectomy), have since been challenged – it is now thought that there is no difference between the two types. However, regarding the type of HRT used after a subtotal hysterectomy, if the main part of your uterus has been removed but the cervix retained, it is currently uncertain whether HRT can be given in the form of oestrogen only or oestrogen combined with progestogen. The slight concern of using oestrogen-only HRT is that there may be some of the cells of the lining of the uterus in the cervical canal, which could become thickened from the oestrogen. This thickening can be prevented by adding in progestogen. To find out if progestogen is required, you may be asked to use oestrogen combined with cyclical progestogen for 3 months after your operation. If there is monthly bleeding during this time, it means that cells are present that are responding to the hormones, so oestrogen and progestogen should be used thereafter. (These hormones can, however, be given together continuously to avoid monthly bleeding.) If there is no bleeding in the first 3 months, then oestrogen can be given on its own thereafter.

6 | Contraception – what to use and when to stop

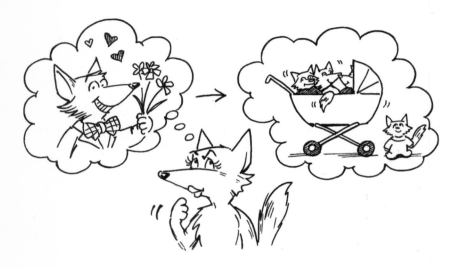

Fertility declines after the age of 35 because of reduced quality of eggs and also because of reduced sexual activity. By the stage of the perimenopause (the time around the menopause), fertility is low though not zero. Pregnancies over the age of 50 are rare but the oldest woman known to have conceived naturally and given birth was aged 57 years. An unplanned pregnancy at an older age can be devastating for the individual woman and can be associated with increased risk of complications such as miscarriage, chromosomal disorders (e.g. Down's syndrome), hypertension and 'gestational' diabetes (diabetes developing during pregnancy).

Women are often unsure how long they should continue using contraception and what type is best at an older age. They often assume, because fertility is low, sexual activity is less frequent and perhaps periods may be becoming infrequent, that contraception is not required. Women in their late reproductive years may also have heavy, irregular or painful periods, which must be taken into account when choosing a method of contraception.

Many women around this stage of life may also be considering the use of hormone replacement therapy (HRT) and wonder if contraception is still needed along with HRT, and if contraception can be used as a form of HRT.

TYPES OF CONTRACEPTION FOR THE OLDER WOMAN

The types of contraception available for older women are the same as those available to younger women and, because of reduced fertility, many of the methods are more effective in the perimenopausal years. No contraceptive method is contraindicated by age alone, though if you smoke, the combined oral contraceptive pill is not recommended after the age of 35.

I'm 43 and my cycle is all over the place after being as regular as clockwork for years. It's so inconvenient, I just don't know when I'm going to come on. I was wondering whether a contraceptive pill might help me?

A low dose contraceptive pill can be used at this stage if you are a non-smoker, not overweight and generally healthy. It would suppress the irregular hormone production from your ovaries and lead to a more regular withdrawal bleed. Some women now continue on the contraceptive pill up until the age of 50. Once you are known to be menopausal, if you wish to continue taking hormone therapy,

HRT is a better option because the hormones used are natural and will be in a lower dose.

Combined oral contraceptive pill

The combined pill is a highly effective method of contraception at all ages and is used by 8% of women over the age of 40. It may have special advantages for older women by helping heavy or painful periods or preventing ovarian cysts. It contains a combination of the two hormones, oestrogen and progestogen, which are given in a high enough dose to suppress ovarian function, preventing egg release. The same hormones are also available now as a patch applied weekly for 3 weeks followed by a patch-free week. Women may continue with the combined pill up to the age of 50 years provided they are fit, slim, non-smokers and have no risk factors for heart disease or stroke, such as high blood pressure, diabetes, or high cholesterol. Non-smokers with no specific risk factors have no increased risk of myocardial infarction (heart attack) with the use of the combined pill at any age. In smokers, it is recommended that the combined contraceptive pill should be stopped at the age of 35 because of the risk of heart disease and stroke. Since the excess risk of heart attack associated with smoking falls 1 year after stopping smoking, and is gone 3–4 years later, women over the age of 35 who have stopped smoking more than 1 year before may consider using the combined pill.

The combined pill must be prescribed by a doctor or prescribing nurse, and blood pressure should be checked regularly. It can be associated with a very slightly increased risk of breast cancer and thrombosis (blood clot), and should not be prescribed for women with migraine or who have had a previous blood clot. The small increased risk of breast cancer is reduced to no excess risk 10 years after stopping.

Using the combined pill in the long term is thought to protect against both cancer of the ovary and of the lining of the womb; a reduction of at least 50% in the risk of ovarian and endometrial cancer with combined pill use has been suggested, and this reduced risk continues for 15 years after stopping.

If I keep taking my contraceptive pill into my late 40s, will it hide any menopausal symptoms I might be having?

The combined contraceptive pill contains high dose, synthetic oestrogen, which suppresses your own ovarian function and masks any symptoms of ovarian failure. Some women notice hot flushes in the week when they don't take the pill when there is a drop in oestrogen level, but the only way to know how your own ovaries are working is to stop the pill for a few months and use some other form of contraception.

I went on to the combined pill when I started a new relationship a year ago. I felt great – years younger with loads more energy, and the problems I'd been having with my lower back vanished overnight. But then I saw a different doctor who said I was too old (I am 49). She put me on a progestogen-only pill and I feel middle-aged and stiff again. Can I persuade her to change her mind?

If you do not smoke, are of normal weight, and do not have significant medical problems, then it would be reasonable to restart the combined pill if it suited you better. The decision should be a joint one between you and your doctor after a full discussion.

The progestogen-only pill ('mini-pill')

The 'mini-pill' is very suitable for older women and there is no upper age limit to using the progestogen-only pill. It is thought to be used by 7% of women aged over 40 years who are using contraception. As it does not contain oestrogen, it can be used by women who are unsuitable for the standard combined contraceptive pill. Therefore, women with problems, such as high blood pressure, migraines, or who have had a previous thrombosis, can use the 'mini-pill'. There is no apparent increase in the risk of heart attack, stroke, blood clot or breast cancer with the 'mini-pill'. Most 'mini-pills' may, however, cause quite erratic periods or cause periods to stop altogether. The 'mini-pill' contains progestogen only and its main contraceptive effect is by causing a thickening of the mucus at the neck of the womb, thereby making it difficult for sperm to travel into the womb.

Recently, a 'mini-pill' has become available which, as well as thickening the mucus, suppresses ovulation in about 97% of women. This can be helpful in women who are beginning to have irregular periods, since some women on this preparation will not have periods at all. The progestogen-only pill must be prescribed by a doctor but can be continued for as long as a woman requires contraception.

Over all ages, the failure rate of the progestogen-only pill is 2–3 pregnancies per 100 women per year but, in women over 40, it is only 0.3 per 100 women per year and so is a very effective choice at this age.

I have really bad migraines at my period time. I'm now 46 and my periods are not as often as they used to be, but I am told that I still need contraception. I couldn't use the contraceptive pill but my doctor has suggested trying a new mini-pill.
I am worried because I always thought that I couldn't take hormones. Is it safe and will it make my migraines worse?

The mini-pill, or progestogen-only pill can be used in people who suffer from migraines and is safe. Migraine that occurs at the time of your periods is probably precipitated by the fluctuation of hormones that happens at this time, with oestrogen and progesterone levels falling just before your period. The newest progestogen-only pill, desogestrel (Cerazette), has been shown to suppress the hormone fluctuations by suppressing ovulation in about 97% of users. In suppressing this fluctuation, it can in fact reduce period-related migraines and can stop periods altogether. It would definitely be worth trying.

Injectable contraception

The 3-monthly progestogen preparation contraceptive injection (medroxyprogesterone acetate – Depo-Provera) is mainly used by young women. It can still be continued up to older ages and is a good treatment for heavy or painful periods and PMS (premenstrual syndrome). There is some current concern that contraceptive injections may increase the risk of osteoporosis in later life by reducing the ovarian production of oestrogen, but any reduction in bone mineral density usually recovers after treatment is stopped. For this reason, many healthcare professionals recommend that women stop Depo-Provera at the age of 45 years to allow return of oestrogen production and recovery of any loss in bone mineral density prior to the menopause. Consideration should also be given to using some other form of contraception if the injection has stopped periods for more than 2 years.

A contraceptive rod (etonogestrel – Implanon) is also available, which is placed under the skin in the upper arm under local anaesthetic. This releases progestogen in a steady level over 3 years. It is an extremely effective contraceptive and does not seem to increase the risk of osteoporosis.

Both the 3-monthly injection and the 3-yearly rod are often chosen because of their convenience.

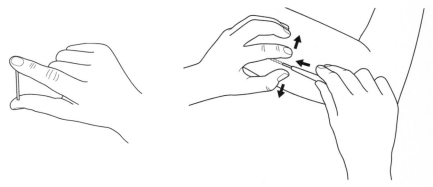

Figure 6.1 Implanon implant (**a**) and being inserted (**b**).

I've been having the Depo-Provera injection for years and it's fantastic because I don't have any periods. Over the last few months, I've been having hot flushes, which are becoming a real nuisance. I'm thinking about using HRT but can I stay on the Depo as well, because I don't want my periods to come back?

It may be that your periods have in fact now stopped anyway but the only way to know would be to stop the Depo injection, use some other form of contraception and see what happens. However, it can sometimes take several months to know whether or not your own hormone production has restarted. Other very effective contraceptives are available and some, such as the hormone-releasing coil, can also reduce bleeding. If you decide to continue the Depo-Provera, then oestrogen could be added in for the flushes. It is very likely that the Depo-Provera will protect the lining of the womb from the possible thickening effect of the oestrogen but it is not licensed for this.

My doctor wants me to come off the 3-monthly Depo injection because she's worried about my bones. I do smoke, although I know I shouldn't because it's bad for my bones as well as everything else it's bad for. I do keep trying to stop but I really want to stay on the injection because it's so easy. I don't want to get pregnant and I know I would never remember to take the pill. Do I really have to stop it?

It has been shown that, if the 3-monthly injection causes periods to stop and is continued for more than 2 years, it may increase a future risk of osteoporosis because it suppresses oestrogen. After 2 years' use, then you should think of having other forms of contraception – there are now many options that are not harmful to your bones. However, if, after discussing the options with your doctor, you feel that the 3-monthly injection is the best for you at this stage, then you can choose to continue, but do reconsider this at a later date, and never give up on trying to stop smoking!

Intrauterine device (IUD or 'coil')

An IUD can be used for contraception at any age. It is very reliable but may cause periods to become heavier or slightly more painful. Having an IUD inserted into the womb is a very minor procedure and, once it is inserted, you do not need to remember anything else for contraception. If an IUD is inserted after the age of 40 years, then it can remain without being changed until the menopause. Although IUDs have not been very widely used over the years in the UK, they are the most common reversible method of contraception worldwide and are becoming much more popular now.

I've had a coil in for 10 years and I'm now 52. My periods stopped 2 years ago. The coil doesn't cause me any problems, so can I just forget about it or should I have it taken out?

The coil should now be taken out. Since your periods stopped 2 years ago, the coil is not needed for contraception any more. Although it may not be causing problems, it could be a source of infection in the future. After the menopause, the canal of the cervix can become narrowed, making it more difficult to remove the coil, so the sooner it is removed the better. If the coil is difficult to remove, it can be helpful to take HRT for a few months, as this can cause some softening of the tissues leading to easier removal.

Intrauterine system (IUS, e.g. Mirena)

The hormone-releasing intrauterine system is a highly effective contraceptive but it also drastically cuts down the amount of bleeding and pain with menstrual periods. It is fitted into the womb like a normal IUD. It is therefore an ideal method for women who have period problems, and can also continue to be used when a woman becomes menopausal and wishes to take HRT. Women should always be warned that there is often a lot of erratic bleeding and spotting in the first few months of use before the bleeding pattern settles down.

Around a quarter of women using this system find that their periods stop altogether.

Mirena, as an example of this system, is licensed for use for contraception for 5 years but, if it is inserted at or after the age of 45, and the bleeding pattern continues to be acceptable, it can be continued to be used for 7 years. However, if it is subsequently used for the progestogen part of HRT, it should be renewed after 4 years.

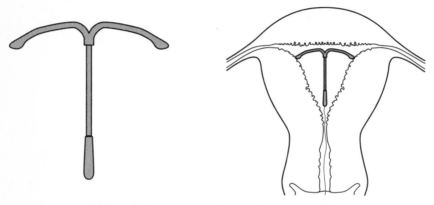

Figure 6.2 Mirena IUD (**a**) and in position (**b**).

I have had a Mirena inserted which has caused my periods to stop. I don't understand where the blood is going – could I be pregnant?

Reducing or stopping bleeding is a common effect of Mirena and, indeed, Mirena is often used for controlling heavy periods. The hormone (progestogen) in the Mirena is released directly into the lining of the womb and makes the lining thin. When it is thin, it is less able to respond to the ovarian hormone stimulation and bleed. Therefore, it's not that the blood is going anywhere else, but that it is not being produced. This can only be a bonus! Mirena is a very effective contraceptive and your chances of pregnancy with Mirena are extremely low.

A few years ago I had a Mirena put in because of heavy periods and because my partner and I were fed up with using condoms. It has been great but now I'm having hot flushes. Can I use HRT along with the Mirena or will it interfere somehow?

It is perfectly OK to take HRT along with having a Mirena device fitted. For women who have not had a hysterectomy, HRT is a combination of oestrogen and progestogen – oestrogen helping to control menopausal symptoms and progestogen to protect the lining of the womb. Since Mirena releases progestogen into the womb, it can be used for the progestogen part of HRT, so that, with a Mirena in place, HRT can be taken as oestrogen-only; this will be simpler than having a combination therapy.

Barrier methods

Condoms are recommended to prevent the spread of sexually transmitted disease, particularly when individuals start a new relationship. They are an effective method of contraception at all ages when used properly. As hormone levels begin to change, many women experience vaginal dryness, which can cause discomfort during intercourse. Vaginal lubricants can be very helpful but care should be taken if oil-based vaginal lubricants are used along with condoms, since some can cause latex condoms to break down and hence reduce the contraceptive effect of the condoms. Diaphragms may be used, often very reliably in older women.

I split up with my husband a few years ago and now I'm in a new relationship. My new partner has had a vasectomy and at 50 I know I'm not fertile anyway, but I wonder if I should still suggest that he uses condoms.

New relationships in later years are becoming more common. Although contraception may not be required, barrier methods such as condoms should still be considered and discussed with your new partner to reduce the risk of sexually transmitted infections. This is discussed in Chapter 12.

Sterilisation

The most commonly used method of contraception by women aged over 40 years is sterilisation, with similar numbers of couples using female sterilisation to those using vasectomy. However, it would rarely be necessary to perform sterilisation in a woman approaching the menopause, since it would not often be justified for someone with low fertility to undergo an invasive surgical procedure when other effective options are available. Despite this, if it is decided that sterilisation is the best option for the couple considered together, then the partner might consider having a vasectomy, since this procedure carries a lower failure rate and less risk compared with female sterilisation.

Over the number of years that sterilisation is used, the failure rate is thought to be 1 in 200 and, if pregnancy does occur after sterilisation, ectopic pregnancy (pregnancy developing outside the womb, e.g. in the tube) can occur. The failure rate following vasectomy is approximately 1 in 2000. Risks of surgery for female sterilisation are increased if the woman has had previous surgery of the abdomen or is overweight, but it is generally quoted as being a complication of surgery in 1 in 200 cases.

I used to take the contraceptive pill until I was sterilised 3 years ago. Since then I've had no end of bother with my periods – they are really heavy and come more often. Could this be due to the sterilisation?

Although periods quite often appear to change after sterilisation, it is unlikely to be directly due to the actual procedure. One explanation is that many women use the oral contraceptive pill for contraception, inducing a regular bleed, which is often lighter than a natural period. Once a woman has been sterilised, she stops taking the pill since it is no longer needed for contraception. The periods then return to whatever is your normal pattern, which was probably heavier and less regular than when you were taking the contraceptive pill.

Another possibility is that hormone changes occur, which affect the period pattern. It has been suggested that sterilisation can affect blood supply to the ovaries, leading to early ovarian decline and hence indirectly to a change in periods, but this association is unclear.

> *I was sterilised 8 years ago when I really thought that I would never want to have any more children, but 2 years later my husband left me; it was the worst time of my life. However, I am now with a wonderful man and we think the world of each other. He's younger than me and has not had any children and, although he is fantastic with my two children from my first marriage, it would be so wonderful if we could have a child together. I'm now 43. Would I be able to have my sterilisation reversed?*

Reversal of sterilisation is rarely available on the NHS and so would have to be funded privately. Unfortunately, the chances of reversal being successful especially with the reduced fertility at your age of 43 would be extremely low. Even the success rate of fertility treatment such as *in vitro* fertilisation (IVF), where eggs are fertilised outside the body, bypassing the fallopian tubes, would probably be only about 5% after the age of 40. It would therefore be unlikely that reversal of sterilisation could be recommended.

Emergency contraception

Emergency hormonal contraception (Levonelle) uses high dose progestogen and has very few contraindications. It can be used at any age if it is thought to be necessary and can be obtained in pharmacies without prescription. It should be taken as a single dose (1500 mcg) within 72 hours of the episode of unprotected intercourse, but ideally as soon as possible.

Natural methods

Natural methods of contraception include using indicators of changes in cervical mucus or body temperature to predict ovulation and then avoiding having sexual intercourse, or using barrier methods during the fertile period, or using the withdrawal method. In the perimenopause, the menstrual cycle is often irregular and body temperature can be variable. Therefore it can be very difficult to work out when the fertile time is. Natural methods are therefore thought to be unreliable with erratic ovulation and irregular periods, and are not recommended at this stage. The withdrawal method is associated with a high failure rate and is not recommended as a reliable method of contraception at any age.

Hormone replacement therapy

It is very important to realise that HRT is not a method of contraception and if a woman's periods have not yet stopped when she starts HRT, then she must use a method of contraception in addition. We know that occasionally women do become pregnant whilst taking HRT if they do not use additional contraception. Methods of contraception to consider using with HRT are: condoms, a diaphragm, an IUD, an intrauterine system or the 'mini-pill'.

WHEN TO STOP CONTRACEPTION

Generally, it is recommended that contraception should be continued until ovulation no longer occurs. This means that contraception should be continued for at least 1 year after your last period if they stopped after the age of 50, and for 2 years if your periods stopped before the age of 50. Once HRT has been started, it can be very difficult to know when contraception can be stopped, since HRT will often produce regular monthly bleeds. It is therefore impossible to know when a woman's natural periods would have stopped. The easiest answer is often just to continue contraception along with HRT until the age of 55 years, at which time it can be assumed that a woman has no further risk of pregnancy; at the age of 55 years, 95.9% of women will be post-menopausal.

I'm 49 and still taking the combined pill; it suits me really well. How do I know when I can stop it? Would a blood test be helpful?

While you are taking the combined pill you cannot know whether or not you are menopausal and blood tests to measure hormone levels are unreliable while you are taking this pill. If you do not have other medical problems and you are of normal weight and don't smoke, you can continue the combined pill up to the age of 50 but it is recommended to stop then. Other contraceptive methods such as barrier methods or the progestogen-only pill should then be considered. If barrier methods are used, they should be continued until you have had 1 year of no periods at which time the menopause can be diagnosed and contraception stopped.

I've been on the mini-pill for years and for the last 2 years I've had no bleeding at all. Does that mean that I'm now into the menopause and can I stop it?

The absence of periods while taking hormonal contraception is not a reliable indicator of menopause and hence does not mean that the mini-pill, or progestogen-only pill, can be stopped. The progestogen-only pill can be continued up to the age of 55 when natural fertility may be assumed to be extremely low. Unlike with the combined pill, while you are on the progestogen-only pill, a blood test to measure follicle stimulating hormone (FSH) can be taken. If FSH is over 30 IU/litre on two occasions more than 1 to 2 months apart, then it can be assumed that your menopause has occurred and you should then continue with contraception for a further year.

7 | Diet, exercise, lifestyle and general health

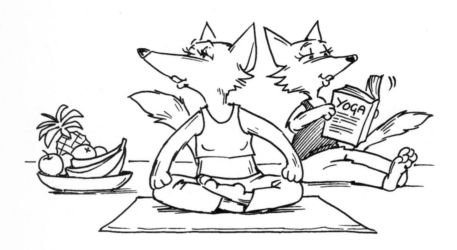

The changes that happen around the time of the menopause often serve as a 'wake up' call; for many years, women with busy lives have often paid little attention to their own health, prioritising their family and work in front of themselves. As hormone levels change and symptoms appear, women will probably seek medical help. The tendency may then be to consider specific treatments to alleviate the symptoms. For many women, treatments can be very effective with minimal risk. However, attention should also be paid to diet and lifestyle; it is often overlooked how important some simple changes can be, not only in reducing menopausal symptoms but also in improving general health and reducing the risk of long-term disease.

DIET

A varied, healthy diet, combined with exercise, is important at all ages, particularly as current estimates suggest that 20% of the adult population in the UK is obese. Obesity is well known to increase the risk of heart disease, type 2 diabetes, gallbladder disease, high blood pressure, osteoarthritis, low back pain, and cancer of the breast, womb and colon. At the menopause, with falling oestrogen levels, along with the ageing effect, energy metabolism is altered leading to increased deposition of fat, particularly around the abdomen, and reduced lean body mass. During adult life, energy requirements reduce by 2% per decade. Therefore, even if the same diet and exercise are followed as in previous years, weight gain and change in body shape will often occur along with the menopause; no change in lifestyle leads to an increase in weight every year of 1–1.5 kg or 10–15 kg each decade. The menopause is therefore the ideal time to make changes and enjoy the benefits!

I've battled with my weight all my life. Now I've hit the menopause and am considering using HRT but am terrified that I'll put even more weight on.

Many women fear weight gain with HRT and often blame HRT for weight gain. In fact studies have shown either no difference in weight gain in women taking HRT compared with those not taking HRT, or even less weight gain in women taking HRT compared with placebo. There is some evidence that HRT can increase lean body mass, reduce abdominal fat and reduce total fat. There are more questions on this aspect in Chapters 3 and 8.

I can't believe how much weight I've put on over the last year.
I used to be able to eat anything and my weight stayed the
same. It's all round my middle – is this middle-age spread?

The change in metabolism with age and, separately, with the menopause, often leads to deposition of fat around the middle, known as 'middle-age' spread or 'midriff'. An increase in abdominal fat distribution (an increase in the waist/hip ratio) has been shown to increase the risk of heart disease. Change in diet combined with increased exercise can control this and lead to significant health benefits. See the questions below in this chapter for more advice on this.

I have had both ovaries removed, and I am not allowed HRT.
Someone told me that oestrogen is also produced by fat and
that is why women lay down some fat around the middle at
the time of the menopause. I am slightly overweight but need
that oestrogen! Should I be dieting in the circumstances?

Oestrogen can be produced in fatty tissue from androgens but not necessarily enough to counteract the effects of the menopause. Unfortunately, it is not a reason to ignore weight gain! You should aim to achieve a weight at which you feel comfortable by general healthy eating and exercise.

What's the best diet to follow – Atkins, soup, cereal diets?
There are so many you hear about, I don't know what to do!

A healthy diet should firstly and most importantly be something that you can stick to and enjoy! There is no point in following a fashionable diet that really doesn't suit you, your budget or your lifestyle. Although some diets claim successful rapid weight loss, an overall change leading to gradual, sustained weight loss of perhaps 1–2 pounds per week and then, when the target weight has been achieved, keeping to a steady weight, is much preferred. Many women find it best to join a slimming club and many are available in most towns but also online. The personal input, advice and motivation may be needed but some women prefer to go it alone. Rather than looking at the problem as a need for a 'diet', we should think of our food as an important part of life, not only in terms of health benefits of correct caloric and nutrient content, but also in relation to social aspects in the preparation of food and enjoyment of social interactions around the table. Many family issues can be resolved around the table during a meal, not with a meal on your knee in front of the television!

Some general principles to follow include:

- eating regularly
- trying not to 'skip' meals
- always making time for breakfast
- trying as much as possible to 'cook from scratch' using fresh foods
- avoiding convenience and refined foods (although they can be very handy at times!)
- using foods with a low glycaemic index (see below)
- cutting down on additives, salt, sugar and caffeine
- avoiding highly calorific foods, and
- eating five portions of fruit and vegetables per day.

Food groups

The important food groups to consider when you are planning a food programme are:

- fats
- carbohydrates
- proteins

- vitamins and minerals, and antioxidants.

Foods that may help against osteoporosis developing are considered in Chapter 4.

Fat

Fat content of food is particularly important at the menopause because it has been shown that an increase in total cholesterol and low density lipoprotein cholesterol occurs at the menopause. Increase in cholesterol leads to an increased risk of heart disease and stroke, cardiovascular disease being the major cause of death in women after the menopause. Diets low in *saturated fat* can decrease the risk of heart disease. Saturated fats are often present in red meat, cheese, butter, cream and eggs, so these foods should be eaten in moderation. *Unsaturated fats*, however, are known to provide benefits, and omega fatty acids in particular have been shown to be beneficial for the cardiovascular system. Omega-6 oils are found in unrefined corn, sesame and sunflower oils. Oily fish is a good source of omega-3 oils and it is recommended that a portion of oily fish should be eaten once or twice per week. Omega-3 oils are also found in linseed oil, pumpkin seeds, walnuts and dark green vegetables.

Carbohydrates

Carbohydrates make up a large part of the western diet: they are filling, easy and inexpensive. Refined carbohydrates found in white and brown sugar, chocolate, cakes, biscuits and sweets provide a rapid rise in your blood glucose level because of rapid digestion. This rise is followed by an equally rapid drop, which can lead to tiredness, feeling low, irritability and sometimes sweating; these symptoms, similar to those that can be experienced in the menopause, can produce an additive effect. Unrefined carbohydrates with a low glycaemic index will provide a steady release of sugar, preventing the rapid rises and falls in levels. Unrefined, complex carbohydrates, which release sugar slowly and should therefore be chosen in preference to refined, simple carbohydrates, are listed in Box 7.1. The glycaemic index was developed in 1980 – it shows the various rates at which carbohydrates break down and release glucose into the bloodstream. The faster the food breaks down, the higher the rating on the index, which sets sugar at 100 and scores all other foods against that number. Some supermarkets are now labelling their foods so that you can see which have a lower GI score.

I get really low in the middle of the morning and feel desperate for a bar of chocolate or biscuits – it's my worst time. What healthy snacks would you recommend?

Firstly, eating a breakfast consisting of a whole grain cereal or porridge would provide a slow release of sugar so that you'd be less likely to get the mid-morning cravings. However, healthy snacks are available: try oatcakes, rice cakes or a banana, or any other fruit. Some chocolate or biscuits are allowed though, but in moderation!

Box 7.1 DIETARY SOURCES OF UNREFINED COMPLEX CARBOHYDRATES

- Basmati rice
- Chickpeas
- Haricot beans
- Kidney beans
- Lentils
- Malt loaf
- Oats (porridge is a great way to start the day)
- Pasta
- Vegetables, particularly sweet potatoes
- Whole grain bread

A friend has mentioned a recipe for an HRT cake. It contains lots of seeds such as linseed. Would this be a good substitute for taking HRT tablets?

Various recipes for HRT or menopause cakes and some commercially available cakes and bread are available, which some women might find beneficial. However, scientific information on effects of these cakes compared with placebo (inactive ingredients) is not available. The content of active ingredients will vary immensely and it is unclear how much you would need to take to achieve any effect. The cakes often contain sources of naturally occurring oestrogens (phytoestrogens). We learn more about phytoestrogens in Chapter 10. It is unlikely that eating a piece of HRT cake would be a good substitute for taking HRT.

Proteins

Proteins are necessary for the formation of bones, muscle, hair and skin, but should preferably be consumed from foods low in saturated fats. You should therefore preferably eat fish, chicken (without the skin), low-fat dairy products, nuts, seeds, grains and beans and eat red meat in moderation.

Vitamins and minerals, and antioxidants

Most women taking a healthy well-balanced diet obtain sufficient vitamins and minerals required and dietary sources are the best way to make sure you are getting a variety. Therefore, for most women, there is no need to take supplements. However, many women nowadays have hectic lifestyles and do not always get everything they need from their diets on a daily basis – this is especially true when women are trying to lose weight, perhaps avoiding some essentials in their diets. Some vegetarians can also be at risk of not obtaining enough nutrients in their diets. Some of our western world diets are deficient in some minerals, not just because we do not eat the right foods, but also because the food growing and processing techniques mean that the food is not as good a quality as it used to be. Consequently, some people choose to take vitamin and mineral supplements which, although helpful for some groups, can be harmful if taken in excess.

Vitamin D is particularly important for menopausal women since it is required to maintain bone health by helping the body to absorb calcium. It is made in the skin from the action of sunlight, and lack of sunlight because of poor climate, being housebound, or being covered up when outside, often leads to a deficiency of vitamin D, particularly in elderly people. Dietary sources include oily fish, dairy products and margarine: two main course portions of oily fish per week are recommended.

Calcium. During the menopause, an adequate daily calcium intake is especially important to help protect and maintain bone density, as bone loss accelerates. Supplements of calcium and vitamin D can be taken if the recommended amount is not achieved but the body copes best with a dietary source of calcium (see Table 7.1). The recommended daily intake of calcium in the UK is 700 mg, but 1200 mg is required if osteoporosis has been diagnosed. Milk and milk products are good sources of calcium, as are cereals (which are often fortified with calcium), dark green leafy vegetables, dried fruits, nuts, seeds and tofu.

Antioxidants, vitamins C and E, selenium and **beta-carotene** are thought to protect the body from damage from chemicals produced as part of the ageing process. Fruits and vegetables provide a range of antioxidants and, rather than identifying sources of specific antioxidants, it is recommended to include at least five portions of fruit and vegetables daily, and to include a wide range of products, to provide different benefits.

Caffeine

Caffeine acts as a stimulant and is enjoyed worldwide with, for most consumers, little harm. However, if taken in excess, it can:

- act as a diuretic causing frequent trips to the loo
- affect sleep

Table 7.1 CALCIUM-RICH FOODS [1]

Food	Quantity	Calcium (mg)*
Dairy products		
Cheese: Camembert	3½ oz/100 g	235
Cheese: Cheddar	3½ oz/100 g	739
Cheese: Cottage	3½ oz/100 g	127
Cheese: Edam	3½ oz/100 g	795
Cheese: low fat (hard)	3½ oz/100 g	840
Cream: double	3½ oz/100 g	49
Cream: single	3½ oz/100 g	91
Cream: whipping	3½ oz/100 g	58
Custard from powder	3½ oz/100 g	140
Fromage frais: fruit	3½ oz/100 g	86
Ice cream: dairy	3½ oz/100 g	100
Ice cream: non-dairy	3½ oz/100 g	72
Milk: semi-skimmed	100 ml	120
Milk: skimmed	100 ml	122
Milk: soya ***	100 ml	89
Milk: whole	100 ml	188
Rice pudding	3½ oz/100 g	88
Yoghurt: fruit	3½ oz/100 g	122
Yoghurt: fruit low-fat	3½ oz/100 g	140
Fish		
Pilchards in tomato sauce	3½ oz/100 g	250
Salmon: tinned	3½ oz/100 g	91
Sardines in oil	3½ oz/100 g	500
Sardines in tomato sauce	3½ oz/100 g	430
Tuna in oil: tinned	3½ oz/100 g	12
Whitebait: fried	3½ oz/100 g	860
Vegetables		
Curly kale: boiled	3½ oz/100 g	150
Okra: stir-fried	3½ oz/100 g	220
Spinach: boiled	3½ oz/100 g	160
Spring greens: boiled	3½ oz/100 g	75
Watercress	3½ oz/100 g	170

Food	Quantity	Calcium (mg)*
Pulses, beans & seeds		
Baked beans	3½ oz/100 g	53
Green/French beans	3½ oz/100 g	56
Red kidney beans	3½ oz/100 g	71
Sesame seeds	3½ oz/100 g	670
Tahini (sesame paste)	3½ oz/100 g	680
Tofu: steamed ***	3½ oz/100 g	510
Cereal products		
Muesli: Swiss-style	3½ oz/100 g	110
Ready Brek	3½ oz/100 g	1200
Special K	3½ oz/100 g	70
White bread **	3½ oz/100 g	177
Wholemeal bread	3½ oz/100 g	106
Fruit		
Apricots: dried	3½ oz/100 g	73
Figs: dried	3½ oz/100 g	250
Currants	3½ oz/100 g	93
Mixed peel	3½ oz/100 g	130
Olives in brine	3½ oz/100 g	61
Oranges	3½ oz/100 g	47
Convenience foods		
Cornish pasty	3½ oz/100 g	60
Lasagne: frozen	3½ oz/100 g	73
Macaroni cheese	3½ oz/100 g	170
Omelette: cheese	3½ oz/100 g	287
Pizza: cheese & tomato	3½ oz/100 g	210
Quiche: cheese & egg	3½ oz/100 g	262
Sausages: low-fat grilled	3½ oz/100 g	130

[1] Ref: McCance and Widdowson's *The Composition of Foods*, 6th summary edition, 2002. Compiled by The Food Standards Agency and Institute of Food Research.

* Please note that the calcium contents (with the exception of milk and bread), have been calculated per 100 g and not on portion sizes. This has been done to make comparisons between various foods easier.

** May be calcium-enriched

*** Different products vary considerably

- contribute to irritability
- perhaps worsen menopausal flushes
- have a possible detrimental effect on bone density.

A cup of instant coffee contains about 66 mg of caffeine, filtered coffee containing more. What is often not realised is that tea also contains caffeine; about 50 mg per cup and many fizzy drinks have high caffeine content.

I really enjoy a cup of tea first thing in the morning – in fact I can't start the day without one, and I take a few cups of coffee during the day. I've now heard that too much caffeine is bad for my bones. How much is too much?

There is no clear guidance on how much caffeine is 'too much', but three or four cups of tea or coffee per day is unlikely to be harmful and, in fact, there is some evidence that tea contains antioxidants, which can be beneficial. If you were taking one cup after another then it would be worth cutting down.

I know that I drink too much coffee – about 10 mugs per day. I've decided that I really should stop but can I just stop completely?

If you are having a high caffeine intake, then you should cut down gradually; sudden withdrawal can lead to headaches, dizziness and shaking. Gradually reduce the amount over a number of weeks. If you need to drink something, substitute with water, fruit juices, herbal drinks or decaffeinated drinks.

Alcohol

Alcohol has become a regular component of the diet in the western world. Research has suggested that low doses can provide benefits for the cardiovascular system, but excess can cause liver damage, increase the risk of osteoporosis, and it may worsen menopausal symptoms. Recommended 'safe' limits are 14 units per week for women (21 for men); women are more susceptible to the toxic effect of alcohol than men. Alcohol has a fairly high calorie content; about 100 calories per glass of wine and 200 calories per glass of beer so, if taken in excess, it can contribute to the problem of weight gain.

Remember also that drinking more than 2–3 units of alcohol per day is thought to increase the risk of breast cancer.

EXERCISE

Whatever diet is followed, weight loss can only be maintained and maximum benefits be enjoyed if a healthy diet is combined with regular exercise. There is no doubt that regular exercise provides huge health benefits and improves wellbeing, yet so many of us fail to give exercise a high priority in our busy lives. It has been estimated that only 25% of women exercise on a regular basis. Exercise can reduce the risks of heart disease, diabetes, stroke, osteoporosis, high blood pressure and depression, and also reduce menopausal flushes. Physical activity improves function and efficiency of the heart muscle, as well as increasing insulin sensitivity and reducing harmful triglycerides, both effects leading to a reduced risk of heart attack.

Weight-bearing exercise such as walking, jogging, running, dancing, tennis and badminton is helpful for maintaining bone density; exercise also benefits the bones by improving muscle tone and strength, hence reducing the risk of falling. The 'wake-up call' brought about by changes at the menopause should lead us to take exercise more seriously and build it into our daily lives.

I've hardly taken any exercise for the last 20 years. Where on earth do I start?

Walking is probably the easiest, simplest form of exercise that does not require anything technical, just a good pair of shoes! Simple changes that can easily be included in your daily routine are a good starting point. For example, you could park your car in the furthest away corner of the car park to try to increase your daily steps. When going up to the first floor, always use the stairs rather than taking the lift and when appropriate try to go to the top floor and then back down. It only takes a few minutes and does make a difference. Any walking is good; you may be happy to walk alone or take a friend with you.

Taking up a sport can suit some women and the competitive aspect may add extra motivation; many women prefer to join a gym where guidance can be given on the type of exercise to start with and how to build up gradually. If you are not used to exercising, you shouldn't launch into strenuous exercise without supervision. Whatever you choose, find something that can be continued regularly, that suits your budget, is not boring and most of all gives you enjoyment.

How often should I exercise? Does it have to be every day and, at 60, am I not too old to start exercising?

Ideally 30 minutes of exercise three to five times per week would be beneficial and it's never too late to increase physical activity. Exercise needs to be adapted to what you are capable of and achievable goals should be set; it would be totally inappropriate to suggest that someone who simply wants to improve their health should follow a training programme of a potential athlete!

Pelvic floor exercise

The pelvic floor muscles can benefit from exercise too to help maintain a good bladder function and control, and also to help towards

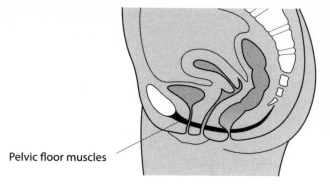

Figure 7.1 Pelvic floor muscles.

enjoyable sexual activity, yet often these very important muscles are forgotten and neglected. Changes associated with the fall in oestrogen levels at the menopause often worsen the function of these muscles – this may be the time when symptoms of poor function are noticed for the first time, such as passing urine often and difficulty controlling urine flow with leakage (particularly when coughing, laughing, sneezing, running or rushing to go to the toilet). The pelvic floor muscles consist of a 'sling'-like sheet of muscles attached between the pelvic bones, helping control bladder and bowel function.

I notice that, now I am 58, I often 'leak' a bit when I am laughing. It's not normally a problem, but, when it does happen, it can be embarrassing. Is there anything I can do to help this problem?

If you are having a lot of problems with bladder control (called stress incontinence in this sort of case), then you should seek specialist help and, with increased awareness of how common the problem is, many health professionals are now specially trained in this area. However, in your case, where this happens only sometimes, the following simple exercises (often called Kegel exercises) can be practised by all women, and probably should be, to prevent problems in the future. Studies have shown that these exercises can cure 50–80% of people with stress incontinence.

1. While sitting or lying with knees a little apart, focus on your pelvic floor and lift and squeeze the muscles both at the front and the back. Try to hold the contraction for at least 3 seconds. As the muscle tone improves, you will gradually be able to hold the contraction for longer.

2. Relax for the same amount of time and then repeat the exercise for as many times as possible, aiming for 10.

3. Next, try short, fast squeezes for the same number of times. These exercises should be repeated daily and if possible, three to four times per day.

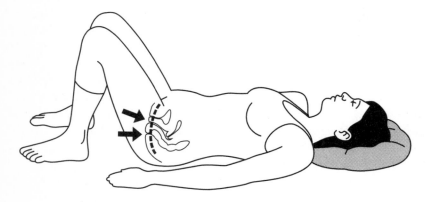

Figure 7.2 Pelvic floor muscle exercises.

How on earth can I fit in walking, relaxing and now pelvic floor exercises as well as everything else in my life?

Many women do have very busy lives and will frequently put work and family first. However, using this time to take stock and invest time in yourself can pay huge dividends in the future. The good news is that pelvic floor exercises can be done while you are sitting at a desk, watching television, sitting in the car at traffic lights, in a meeting or when talking on the phone; therefore they should not take up any extra time!

SMOKING

Smoking has many well-known adverse effects, such as increasing the risk of cancer, emphysema, heart disease and stroke, but also it has specific effects on the menopause. Women who smoke have been shown to have an earlier age of menopause than non-smokers, and smoking has been shown to increase the risk of osteoporosis; it has been suggested that smoking can reduce bone mass by up to 25%. Skin wrinkles, which are common at the menopause, are increased by smoking because of a disruptive effect on collagen in skin and other tissues. Further, women who smoke and take HRT often find that the tablet form of HRT is not very effective in controlling symptoms, and research has shown that tablet HRT does not improve bone density nor lower cholesterol in the same way as it does in non-smokers. It therefore seems that smoking affects hormone production and modifies the effect of tablet HRT, so it may be reasonable to suggest that, for women who smoke and wish to take HRT, non-tablet forms of HRT should be used, such as a patch or gel. Of course the ideal solution would be to stop smoking but, although much more help and support is now available for those who wish to stop smoking, for many this will be a very difficult option.

Can nicotine patches interfere with HRT patch or gel therapy?

The nicotine patch works by delivering small, controlled doses of nicotine into the bloodstream without the other toxic chemicals that are present in cigarette smoke. Several dosage strengths are available and the dosage is gradually reduced until the patch is no longer required. It can affect the way that some medicines work, and it should not be used if you have had a recent heart attack or stroke, or if you have worsening angina or irregular heart rhythm. Be careful also if you have thyroid disease, diabetes, high blood pressure, kidney or liver disease, skin rashes or skin disease. You should not smoke while using nicotine replacement, since an overdose of nicotine may occur. It is very unlikely that nicotine patches would interfere with HRT patches or gel. Since there may be some burning, itching or tingling at the site of the nicotine patch, especially within the first hour of applying it, and skin redness may occur, the nicotine patch and HRT patch or gel should not be applied to the same area.

RELAXATION

The common modern-day problem of stress can affect how you feel and how you cope with the menopause. Because stress is difficult to measure, research on the role of stress and menopausal symptoms is lacking, but we have certainly seen many women whose symptoms have been reduced when a stressful situation is resolved. Of course, we rarely have the answer to the difficulties in which many of us find ourselves, and it seems that domestic problems often coincide with the time of the menopause; as our hormones are deserting us, we may also have teenage children doing what teenagers do, elderly relatives needing help, and partners having a mid-life crisis, to name but a few issues! At this time then, perhaps more than any other, it is vital to learn how to switch off and relax. For some, that may mean being pampered at a luxurious spa occasionally, but for most of us, simpler methods such as a candlelit bath, listening to music, reading a book, going for a walk, going to yoga classes, or taking up a hobby can be very effective. Make time for yourself and you will then be more able to look after others! See the *Techniques* section in Chapter 10.

BREAST AWARENESS AND SCREENING

It is important for all women to be 'breast aware' which means look-ing out for any changes in the way that your breasts look or feel and reporting any concerns to your doctor or nurse (Box 7.2). Currently in the UK, all women aged between 50 and 70 years are offered breast screening every 3 years by mammography. A mammogram is an X-ray of the breast, which can enable health professionals to detect breast changes, which may be due to cancer.

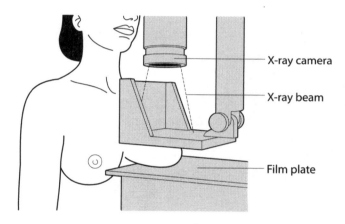

Figure 7.3 The mammogram being taken.

My mum had breast cancer when she was only 45. I'm worried about waiting until I'm 50 to have a check. Would I be able to have screening sooner?

If you have a family history of breast cancer, it can be discussed with your doctor. From your family history, it can be worked out if you are thought to be at high risk of breast cancer and, if so, earlier screening can be arranged.

Box 7.2 BREAST SELF-AWARENESS AND EXAMINATION*

To be breast aware you should become familiar with your own breasts. Understand how they may change at different times during the month – size and feel can change before or just after a period. Pregnancy, age, HRT and menopause will all affect the size and feel of your breasts.

Step 1: Start by looking at your breasts in the mirror – keep your shoulders straight and your arms on your hips. Your breasts should be:

- their usual size, shape, and colour, i.e. usual *for you*
- evenly shaped without visible distortion or swelling.

If you see any of the following changes, go and see your doctor as soon as possible:

- change in shape or size of breast or nipple
- nipple discharge
- dimpling, puckering, scaling, discolouration or bulging of the skin
- a nipple that has changed position or an inverted nipple (pushed inward instead of sticking out)
- redness, soreness, rash, or swelling.

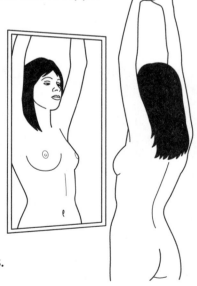

Step 2: Raise your arms and look for the same changes.

Step 3: Feel your breasts while you are lying down:

- Use your right hand to feel your left breast and then your left hand to feel your right breast. Use a firm, smooth touch with the first few fingers of your hand, keeping your fingers flat and together.

- Go over your whole breast from top to bottom, side to side – from your collarbone to the top of your abdomen, and from your armpit to your cleavage.

- Follow a regular pattern to make sure that you have covered the whole breast. For example, begin at the 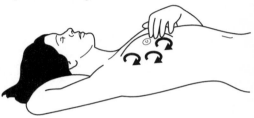 nipple, and move in ever increasing circles until you reach the outer edge of you breast. Move your fingers up and down vertically, in rows, making sure that you feel all the breast tissue: first just beneath your skin with a soft touch, and down deeper with a firmer touch down to your ribcage.

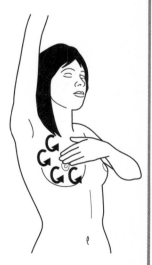

Step 4: Finally, feel your breasts while you are standing or sitting. Many women find that the easiest way to feel their breasts is when their skin is wet and slippery, so they like to do this while in the bath or shower. Cover your entire breast, using the same hand movements described in Step 4.

* Adapted from www.breastcancer.org and http://hosted.aware.easynet.co.uk

Do I need to have a mammogram before I start HRT?

There is no need for a mammogram before starting HRT if you do not have any breast symptoms and, once you are taking HRT, you do not need to have a mammogram any more often than the 3-yearly screening on the National Health, unless any breast problems develop in between times.

When I went for my mammogram, the lady said that my breasts were dense and was I taking HRT? What does this mean and will the mammogram be less accurate because I'm taking HRT?

Some types of HRT, such as oestrogen combined with progestogen rather than oestrogen alone or tibolone, can increase the density of the breast tissue sometimes picked up on a mammogram. It has been suggested that this can make it more difficult to see very early cancers. If the view is not clear, then you may be offered further assessment by more X-rays or an ultrasound scan. It is possible that low doses of HRT that are now recommended as a starting point may not increase breast density as much as higher doses that were often used in the past.

CERVICAL SCREENING

All women in the UK are offered screening in the form of a cervical smear between the ages of 20 or 25 up to 60 or 64, depending on where you live. This simple test is very effective at detecting changes on the cervix (neck of the womb), which may lead to cervical cancer. Treatment of such early changes has hugely reduced the numbers of women developing cervical cancer. It is very important to keep up to date with smears up to, during and after the menopause. Smears do not have to be taken more often if you are taking HRT.

I had a hysterectomy last year but kept my cervix intact.
I now find that I have been deleted from my surgery's list of
patients for cervical smears. Don't I still need screening?

Screening should be continued if the cervix is still present. Discuss this with your doctor and arrange to be put back on the list. Having smears taken is no more difficult following a hysterectomy, and they do not have to be taken any more often than usual.

8 | Hormone replacement therapy (HRT)

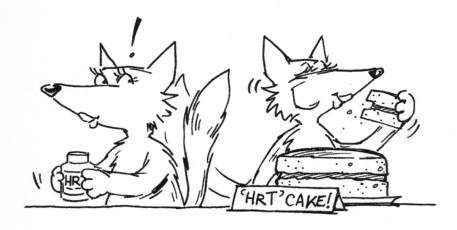

Although HRT has been available for more than 60 years and has been extensively researched, it is still surrounded by controversy. Probably more so today than ever before – both women and health professionals are uncertain about its effects and particularly about its risks. In the 1990s, HRT was taken by millions of women because it was seen as having huge benefits, not only for control of menopausal symptoms but also for protecting against osteoporosis, heart disease and dementia; the known small increased risk of breast cancer with long-term use was overshadowed by the significant benefits. However, use of HRT dropped dramatically in 2002–2004 following the publication of the Women's Health Initiative (WHI) trial and the

Million Women study. Risks associated with HRT as shown by these trials received widespread media attention – the risks were exaggerated, leading to many women stopping HRT, perhaps unnecessarily. Further, the population of women in the WHI trial were quite different, being much older than women who usually take HRT to control menopausal symptoms, and they consequently had different risks. It is regrettable that further analysis of results, particularly of the WHI trial, which showed that the risks of HRT in women in the early menopausal years and in women taking HRT after a hysterectomy are in fact very small and are very likely to be far outweighed by the benefits, has received very little media attention. Shouldn't women be given the whole story? Furthermore, more recent evidence is suggesting that HRT taken in the early menopausal years may in fact be protective against heart disease and dementia as was previously believed – the pendulum continues to swing!

HRT is neither necessary nor appropriate for every woman, yet it is still a very useful treatment. When it is used appropriately, with individualised treatment and regular review for women with risk/benefit balance considered, then for many women the benefits will continue to outweigh the small risks, and HRT should continue to play an important role in menopause management.

WHAT IS HRT?

HRT stands for hormone replacement therapy, which consists mainly of oestrogen. Since many problems associated with the menopause are thought to be due to reduced levels of oestrogen, HRT aims to replace this. It is often now referred to as HT, hormone therapy but, for this book, we will use the better known term of HRT.

Oestrogens

The oestrogens used in HRT are referred to as 'natural' because they resemble substances produced in the body and they include oestradiol, oestrone and oestriol, which are usually made from soya beans or yam extracts. Conjugated equine oestrogens made from horse urine are also sources of the naturally occurring oestrogen, oestrone sulphate. People respond differently to different types, routes and doses of oestrogen, and sometimes several adjustments of therapy are required. If HRT is taken after a hysterectomy, usually oestrogen alone is required (see Chapter 5).

Is all HRT made from horses' urine? I'm allergic to horses so do you think I'd react badly to HRT?

Only one brand of oestrogen is made from horse's urine (conjugated equine oestrogen). If you are allergic to horses, this is probably because you react to their dander; it is unlikely that there would be a problem with the HRT made from their urine. Sometimes different types and routes need to be tried before you find the most suitable for you.

Progestogens

For women in whom the uterus (womb) is present, a progestogen is added to the oestrogen to reduce the risk of oestrogen causing thickening, and eventually cancer, of the endometrium (lining of the womb). Progestogens are mostly made from plant sources and resemble the naturally occurring progesterone, usually produced from the ovary in the second half of the menstrual cycle. The two main types of progestogen currently used in HRT are: those most closely resembling progesterone (drospirenone, dydrogesterone and medroxyprogesterone acetate) and those derived from testosterone (norethisterone, norgestrel and levonorgestrel). The duration and frequency of the progestogen taken determines the presence and pattern of bleeding, and the type used is influenced by presence or absence of periods, and age.

If side effects are experienced on one type, changing the type or route of progestogen may help.

Do I really have to take the progestogen bit of the HRT? I feel really good when I take the white tablets in the first half of the pack but I get bloating and feel quite low on the green tablets for the last 12 days. What would happen if I just missed out the green ones?

If oestrogen alone was given to someone who had **not** had a hysterectomy, i.e. they still have their womb, then, because oestrogen stimulates the lining of the womb, it could increase the risk of thickening of the lining and even cancer of the lining. To reduce this risk, progestogen must also be taken to protect the lining. Many women find that they have side effects with the progestogen part of their HRT and, if this happens, the progestogen can be changed both in type and route (read about side effects later in this chapter).

Can I get HRT for free or do I have to pay privately?

In the UK, HRT has to be prescribed and therefore requires the usual prescription charge. The oestrogen-only and continuous combined preparations incur one charge but, unfortunately, the preparations containing daily oestrogen and progestogen for only part of each monthly pack (sequential therapy) incur a double charge.

HOW TO TAKE HRT

How do I know if I'm getting enough oestrogen – shouldn't I have a blood test?

The usual way by which we know if the dose is correct is by the effect on your symptoms – if these are controlled with no or minimal side effects, then it is likely that the dose is correct. Blood tests can be taken to measure oestradiol levels if there is a poor response to HRT, but are useful only if the oestrogen is in non-tablet form, since tablet oestrogen is converted in the body to products that are not usually measured. Oestradiol measurements are recommended if oestrogen is given by implant, since sometimes, with this form of therapy, very high oestrogen levels can be reached, which must be monitored. It is now known that much lower doses of oestrogen than were used in the past can be used with good symptom control and beneficial effect on bones – in fact it is now recommended that women start with a low dose preparation.

I've been taking HRT for a few years now and it has really helped my flushes but I'm fed up with the 'monthly'. Can I change to one that stops the bleeding?

Period-free HRT can be used if it is fairly sure that your own period cycle has stopped. You would know this if you had at least 1 year without periods before you started HRT, or if you are now aged 54 years or more. If these don't apply and you start period-free HRT when your ovaries are still producing ups and downs of hormones, your own cycle would continue to produce stimulation of the lining of the womb and hence bleeding, which would not be harmful but would be a nuisance. The more sure you are that your own hormone production has stopped, the more likely you are to be able to take period-free HRT without any bleeding.

Routes for HRT

If HRT is required for control of general symptoms such as hot flushes, sweats or insomnia, or for treatment or prevention of osteoporosis, then it should be taken in a way that circulates through your whole body. This is known as systemic HRT. Systemic oestrogen can be taken as a daily tablet, a weekly or twice weekly patch, daily gel, daily nasal spray or a 6-monthly implant. Oestrogen combined with progestogen can be taken by tablet or weekly or twice weekly patch. Progestogen alone can be taken by tablet, vaginal gel or by a progestogen-releasing intrauterine system, such as Mirena. The different routes of oestrogen used have different metabolic effects

Table 8.1 TYPES OF SYSTEMIC HRT

Tablet	Patch	Gel	Nasal spray	Implant
Oestrogen only or oestrogen combined with progestogen. Taken daily	Oestrogen only or oestrogen combined with progestogen. Changed weekly or twice weekly depending on brand	Oestrogen only. Applied once daily. Useful if skin irritation with patches	Oestrogen only. One spray in each nostril once or twice daily. Tends to cause less breast tenderness	Oestrogen only. Small pellet inserted under the skin, usually in lower abdomen. Administered 6-monthly

(e.g. on clotting factors and lipids) but the implications of the differences are controversial and the main factors determining choice of route are individual preference, response and past medical history. Most often, HRT is started in tablet form.

Some factors that contribute to choosing the non-tablet route include:

- individual preference
- poor symptom control with tablet HRT
- side effects from using the tablets, such as nausea
- bowel disorder, which may affect absorption of tablet therapy
- history of migraine (when steadier hormone levels achieved with a patch may be preferable – see later in this chapter about migraines)
- lactose sensitivity (all tablet preparations of HRT contain lactose)
- history of gallstones
- current use of medications such as antiepileptic medication, which may interfere with the break-down of the tablet form
- variable high blood pressure

- high triglyceride levels

- history of venous thrombosis (blood clot)

- liver disease.

My HRT tablets don't seem to work – I still have awful flushes and am so sweaty that I have to change the sheets at night. My friend's tablets are the same as mine and work a treat for her. Why aren't they working for me?

There is a huge variation between women in how much oestrogen is absorbed from the bowel and how quickly it is broken down before it reaches the oestrogen receptors around the body to have an effect. Some people have bowel disorders that can reduce the absorption. Women who smoke are thought to break down their tablet oestrogen quicker than non-smokers, as are those who take certain medications such as some treatments for epilepsy. If a highish dose HRT tablet is ineffective, then trying another route such as a patch might be helpful. Also, it is always also worth looking for other factors such as diet and lifestyle factors (see Chapter 7) and other illnesses or medications (see Chapter 11) that may be contributing to the symptoms.

Patches

I use an HRT patch, which I like, but I get some redness and itchiness on the place where the patch has been. What should I do?

If you are happy with the effect of the patch but not with the skin reaction, then trying a different make of patch may help. If this also causes skin irritation, then an oestrogen gel can provide oestrogen in the same way as the patch but tends to cause less skin irritation. Gels are applied once a day, usually to the thigh or upper arm, but the gels currently available contain only oestrogen. Therefore if you haven't had a hysterectomy and also require progestogen, taking progestogen separately would be recommended.

I've heard about HRT patches. I think I might want to try them since I'm hopeless at remembering tablets, but where would I stick them and do they come off in the bath?

HRT patches should be applied on the hip, thigh, bottom or lower abdomen and, when you are putting on a new one, put it in a different place. They should not be applied near the breasts. Generally, they stay on very well even in the bath or shower and should not need to be taken off beforehand.

Implant

My friend has HRT by implant, with no need to remember any tablets. This sounds nice and easy. Can anyone have one?

The implant is very convenient, since it is administered 6-monthly, but it does require a small procedure by the doctor to put in, and can sometimes produce very high oestrogen levels, which can be difficult to control. Also, if there are problems due to the implant, then it can't be removed and you just have to wait for the effect to wear off, whereas any of the other treatments can easily be stopped if necessary. The implant is oestrogen only so is generally just used for women who have had a hysterectomy. It is particularly useful when there is difficulty controlling symptoms with other types of HRT but it is worth trying other types of HRT before resorting to the implant.

Finding the type of HRT that suits best involves a full discussion of the pros and cons of each and should take into account past history and personal preferences. Sometimes several types need to be tried before getting it right. For the majority of women, the advice about and prescribing of HRT can be carried out by the GP or practice nurse but referral to a specialist clinic may be required if the history is complicated, there is poor response to treatment, there are problems with side effects of treatment, or the GP feels that the topic is outside his or her sphere of knowledge.

WHEN TO TAKE HRT

HRT in the perimenopause

If HRT is commenced in the early stages of ovarian decline when periods are still present (the perimenopause), oestrogen is taken every day and progestogen for 10–14 days per month (sequential HRT). This cyclical progestogen leads to a monthly withdrawal bleed in about 85% of women. There are several types of oestrogen and progestogen, which can be taken in sequential form, and there are tablet and patch preparations. If the periods are becoming infrequent, the progestogen can be taken for 2 weeks every 3 months, leading to a 3-monthly bleed (long-cycle HRT). Currently there is one tablet form of long-cycle HRT available.

HRT in the post-menopause

If you haven't had a period for more than 1 year (post-menopause) before starting HRT, or you are aged 54 or more, progestogen can be taken every day along with the oestrogen (continuous combined HRT). Continuous combined, or period-free, HRT may cause some bleeding in the first 6 months, but should not cause bleeding thereafter. Continuous combined HRT causes the lining of the womb to remain thin instead of going through stages of stimulation and then shedding, as happens in the normal cycle and with sequential therapy. If there is bleeding after you have taken continuous combined HRT for more than 6 months, then you should report this to your doctor and an investigation will be arranged.

Several types of oestrogen and progestogen are available in both tablet and patch in the continuous combined form. Also used in the post-menopause is tibolone (Livial), a tablet with oestrogenic, progestogenic and androgenic properties. Because of its androgenic component (like the male hormone, testosterone), tibolone can be particularly helpful for reduced libido. Current evidence suggests

that tibolone does not increase breast density as seen on mammo-
grams, which may occur with other types of HRT, but long-term use
of tibolone is thought to be associated with a similar slightly
increased risk of breast cancer to that of oestrogen alone, though
this is less than that of oestrogen plus progestogen.

Does it matter if I forget to take my HRT tablets? Do I then have to take extra?

Missing a few tablets is not a disaster and quite often happens. If
you are taking oestrogen only, you may notice some symptoms
such as hot flushes returning but that is all and they should settle
again when the tablets are restarted. If you have not had a hysterectomy and are taking oestrogen combined with progestogen, then
missing some could also cause a little irregular bleeding, which
should also settle when the tablets are restarted. It is not necessary to
take extra tablets to make up for the missed ones, just continue taking one tablet per day. If forgetting a daily tablet is a recurring
problem, then another route of HRT, such as a patch, would be
worth considering.

How long can I take HRT for?

This must be the question that I am most often asked! As long as
you understand why you are taking HRT and have weighed up
the risks and benefits (see later sections in this chapter), then really
you can take HRT for as long or as short a time as you wish. The
main reason that women choose to take HRT is for control of their
menopause symptoms and, because we can never predict how long
symptoms will go on for, we cannot predict how long treatment is
required for. We do recommend having a trial off HRT every 2–3
years to see if symptoms are still present; it is the only way that you
will know whether or not you are still benefiting from the treatment.
The main risk with taking HRT for more than 5 or 10 years after the
age of 50 is a small increased risk of breast cancer and that has to be

weighed against benefits (see later section). The balance is very individual and, although others can advise you what to do, only you can make the decision.

What check-ups do I need before starting HRT?

Make sure that you have an assessment of your general health – this will include information on diet and lifestyle, particularly smoking and alcohol intake, a weight check, blood pressure measurement and, if indicated, a cholesterol level assessment. Blood tests to confirm that you have reached the menopause are not necessary, if it is obvious from your history, but it may be worth having your thyroid function checked; thyroid problems are very common and can cause similar symptoms to the menopause. If the menopause is early or premature, then hormone levels should be checked to confirm the diagnosis and to look for an underlying cause.

My doctor wants me to stop my HRT because I've been on it for 5 years. How do I stop it and what will I do if those terrible flushes and sweats come back?

It is a good idea to see how you are without the HRT – you may not need it now! How to stop it depends on what type you are on: if you are taking a medium- or high-dose preparation, then it is worth cutting down to a lower dose for a few months before stopping; if you are already on a low-dose preparation, then it can just be stopped. Preparations that cause a monthly bleed should be stopped at the end of a pack but period-free types can be stopped at any time. When you are having a trial off HRT, try to stay off for at least 3 months before deciding whether or not to restart; symptoms may come back on first stopping, but then often reduce; some women find that they are OK initially but then symptoms gradually come back. If menopausal symptoms do return and persist, they may not be as bad as before the HRT was started, and some women choose to cope without any treatment, or may try alternative therapies (see

Chapters 7 and 10). For some, the symptoms will be as bad as ever and, if other treatments don't help, your doctor might suggest that you restart HRT and then try stopping again in the future.

What check-ups do I need while I'm taking HRT?

When you start on HRT therapy, or change to a new type, book up to see your GP or practice nurse after 3 months to assess how effective the treatment has been, whether you have had any side effects and the type needs to be changed, and also to measure blood pressure. Once settled on a treatment, you should have a check-up at least once a year to discuss the effect of treatment, to measure your blood pressure and to talk about balancing benefits and risks of ongoing treatment. In between visits, you should contact a health professional if you have any problems such as irregular bleeding, side effects, recurrence of symptoms or other medical problems.

HRT FOR MENOPAUSAL SYMPTOMS

The two current licensed indications for prescribing HRT are:

- relief of menopausal symptoms
- prevention/treatment of osteoporosis.

Systemic HRT can be very effective in relieving symptoms such as hot flushes, sweats, mood swings, irritability, insomnia, palpitations, joint aches, vaginal dryness and discomfort and urinary frequency. Many trials have shown that HRT can reduce symptoms such as flushes and sweats by up to 77% compared with *placebo* (an inactive compound) and, currently, HRT is still the most effective treatment available.

For the vaginal and bladder symptoms, vaginal oestrogen alone can be used. If HRT is taken for symptom relief only, then your doctor will advise stopping the HRT every 2 to 3 years to determine whether or not treatment is still required. If symptoms return, HRT can be restarted after discussing the pros and cons with you. The dose of HRT for symptom control should be the lowest dose of oestrogen that controls symptoms, starting with a low dose preparation and increasing the dose if necessary after 3 months.

If you have poor symptom control with HRT:

- allow 3–6 months on therapy to ensure full effect

- increase dose or change from tablet to non-tablet form if the oestrogen dosage is inadequate

- change to a non-tablet form if a bowel disorder leads to poor absorption

- increase your tablet dose or change to a non-tablet route if other drugs you are taking are causing interaction problems, e.g. barbiturates, phenytoin or carbamazepine

- change the delivery system if you have poor patch adhesion

- ask your doctor if you have been diagnosed correctly – other conditions such as thyroid problems and poor glucose control, and lifestyle factors, can cause similar symptoms to those of the menopause

- you may have unrealistic expectations – HRT can help symptoms owing to oestrogen deficiency but it is not an answer to all our problems!

Doesn't HRT just delay the menopause and won't all my symptoms come back when I stop it?

Many women manage to stop HRT after a few years, or sometimes even after a few months, and find that their symptoms are either much reduced and manageable, or do not come back at all. However, some women do experience symptoms that are as bad as ever when HRT is stopped and may choose to restart it. There is no way of predicting how you are going to respond. It is not clear whether or not HRT simply delays the onset of symptoms and your body has to readjust to the lower hormone levels again when HRT is stopped, or whether HRT controls symptoms while they are present, such that, if they return on stopping, they may well have continued right up until then anyway if HRT had not been taken.

I'd like to go on HRT but my friend tells me that doctors will prescribe it only if you get a lot of hot flushes. I don't get any but I am troubled with stiff joints and my sex life is really suffering because I can't seem to produce any lubrication. I'm sure my husband thinks I've gone off him. Should I tell my doctor I get hot flushes anyway, just to be sure I will get the prescription?

HRT can be prescribed for many menopausal symptoms including hot flushes, and other symptoms such as you describe. Just be honest with your doctor – there's no need to make up symptoms!

Flushes

I use HRT for flushes and it worked really well for a few years but now, despite still taking HRT, the flushes are coming back. Am I becoming immune to the HRT?

Often HRT is started when your ovaries are still producing some oestrogen, and the HRT 'tops up' the levels of oestrogen in your system. Later, your own oestrogen production will decrease further so even though your HRT is the same, the total amount of oestrogen in your system has reduced. This fall in oestrogen level can cause further symptoms. In this case, it is worth trying a different dose or route of HRT. When symptoms return it is also worth remembering that other factors in your life may have changed, such as diet, stress and other medication.

If I take HRT or some other treatment for my flushes, won't they just come back when I stop treatment?

HRT is very effective in controlling menopausal flushes and doesn't necessarily cause them to recur when treatment is stopped. About 25% of women will still have flushes after stopping HRT. The current recommendation is to have a trial off treatment every few years to see if it is still required, whether it be HRT or something else. It is thought that using a low-dose preparation will make it less likely that flushes will return on stopping, but we don't have much scientific evidence to confirm this.

Vaginal symptoms

If oestrogen is required only for vaginal or urinary symptoms, vaginal oestrogen is available in the form of vaginal tablets, creams, pessaries or a vaginal ring.

Table 8.2 TYPES OF HRT FOR VAGINAL SYMPTOMS

Tablet (e.g. Vagifem)	Pessary (e.g. Orthogynest)	Cream (e.g. Ovestin or Orthogynest)	Ring (e.g. Estring)
Small, easy to insert. Has been shown that it can be used for up to 2 years continuously without systemic absorption	Slightly larger than vaginal tablet, easily inserted	Helpful if irritation is on the outer lips, but some women find creams 'messy'	Vaginal ring which remains in place for 3 months and is licensed for up to 2 years' use. Helpful if twice-weekly application inconvenient

I've recently stopped my HRT tablet because of the risk of breast cancer, having taken it for 10 years. My flushes now are not too bad, much less than when I started the HRT, but I'm having awful vaginal dryness with an itch and a burning feeling. I never had any problems when I was on the HRT. Should I go back on it?

This is a common problem and can be very effectively treated with vaginal oestrogen which, if used in the starting dose – nightly for 2 weeks and then twice weekly – does not get absorbed into your system and therefore would not be associated with an increased risk of breast cancer. This would be worth trying first rather than restarting the HRT tablet. There are also non-hormonal vaginal moisturisers available which can be very helpful.

I had a bad reaction to vaginal oestrogen in the past and, after stopping HRT, I have vaginal soreness and bladder infections. How can I be helped?

There are different types of vaginal oestrogen and it may be worth trying a different one. Some women have problems with vaginal oestrogen cream but have been fine with a vaginal oestrogen tablet or pessary. If none of these are suitable, there are non-hormonal vaginal moisturisers, which can be very helpful. These can be bought at pharmacies and one type, ReplensMD, is also now available on prescription.

Osteoporosis

Systemic HRT has also been shown to be beneficial for treatment and prevention of osteoporosis for women who have, or are thought to be at risk of, osteoporosis. Although HRT is not now regarded as the first line of treatment for osteoporosis, it still has a place in the management of osteoporosis, particularly if a woman with osteoporosis also has menopausal symptoms, if she has had a premature or early

Table 8.3 BONE-PROTECTIVE DOSES OF OESTROGEN

Type of oestrogen	Dose
Oral oestrogen	1–2 mg
Oral conjugated equine oestrogen	0.3–0.6 mg
Oestradiol patch	25–50 µg
Oestradiol gel	1–5 g, depending on preparation
Oestradiol implant	50 mg, 6-monthly

menopause (when it is recommended that HRT be taken until the normal age of the menopause), or if other bone-protective treatments have been tried and are not tolerated. See Chapter 4 for more information on menopause and osteoporosis.

Doses of oestrogen that are currently regarded as bone protective are given in Table 8.3.

Over the years it has been found that much lower doses of oestrogen than were previously thought to be required have a beneficial effect on bone.

Other benefits

Other possible benefits of HRT include reduction in the risk of colon cancer, Alzheimer type dementia, cataract formation, dry eyes and macular degeneration. Other women have found improved dentition, skin healing and reduced skin wrinkling. These possible benefits are not currently regarded as indications for HRT and whether or not HRT does provide such benefits is unclear.

I have been on HRT for a year now and I think my skin is so much nicer. Do you think HRT really improves skin?

A recent study seems to confirm that this does occur. Although it was a small study, it did show that women who used HRT had more elastic skin and less severe wrinkling than women who had never used HRT; this was measured by visual assessment of severity of wrinkles and skin rigidity at the cheek and forehead by a plastic surgeon, who was unaware of which of the women had used HRT. It is, however, unlikely that HRT would be given purely for this effect, but it can be an additional benefit for those women who choose to take HRT for menopausal symptom control.

SIDE EFFECTS OF HRT

HRT can cause side effects, which may be due to either the oestrogen or the progestogen part. It is therefore important for your doctor to try to work out which hormone is causing the problems so that your therapy can be adjusted appropriately. Often, a different preparation may be tried that contains exactly the same hormone but made by a different company and sold by a different name. It is important to read the label to check which types of oestrogen and progestogen are involved. With any HRT it is worth continuing for at least 3 months before changing the preparation, since often there may be some side effects initially but these may then settle by 3 months. If not, then a change should be considered.

In women who have not had a hysterectomy, irregular bleeding in the first few months after starting HRT may occur. See your doctor for further assessment if your:

- bleeding on monthly bleed-type therapy becomes heavier, prolonged or irregular

- bleeding persists on period-free therapy beyond 6 months

- bleeding occurs after a spell of no bleeding.

If you do not bleed at all on a monthly bleed-type (sequential) HRT, don't worry! This occurs in about 15% of women on this type and is not abnormal. Investigation is not required and your doctor may suggest changing to a period-free type.

Table 8.4 MANAGEMENT OF SIDE EFFECTS OF HRT

Side effects	*Management*
Oestrogenic Breast tenderness/enlargement Leg cramps Bloating Nausea Headache	*For breast symptoms:* Evening primrose oil, starflower oil, or reduce dose of oestrogen *For gastrointestinal symptoms:* Take with food or change route *Other side effects:* Change type or route
Progestogenic PMS-type symptoms Breast tenderness Lower abdominal pain Backache Depressed mood Acne/greasy skin Headache	**Change progestogen** *Testosterone derived:* Norethisterone, Norgestrol, Levonorgestrel *Progesterone-derived:* Medroxyprogesterone, Dydrogesterone, Drospirenone **Change route** Progestogen by intrauterine system or vaginal gel avoids side effects **Change type of HRT** If postmenopausal, change to continuous combined or tibolone – avoids symptoms of progestogen fluctuation

Headaches and migraines

I had headaches when I was taking the second half of my HRT pack. My HRT was Elleste Duet. My doctor has changed me to Femoston. Will it help my flushes as well and won't it give me the same problems?

Femoston contains the same type of oestrogen as Elleste Duet and therefore should be just as helpful for your flushes. It sounds as though it was the progestogen part of Elleste Duet that was causing the headaches. The progestogen part of Femoston is a different type and so may well suit you better. Women respond differently to different types of both oestrogen and progestogen; many women are well suited to the progestogen in Elleste Duet. Sometimes it takes a few adjustments of therapy to find the best one for you.

I used to have migraines around the time of my periods. When my periods stopped it was wonderful not to have the migraines but the flushes and not sleeping was awful. I was so tired that I struggled to get through each day. I started some HRT tablets – great for flushes and I am now getting a full night's sleep again, but I have started having migraines again. I don't know which is worse!

Migraines can be worsened by fluctuating hormone levels as used to happen around the time of your period. By taking a daily HRT tablet there is some further fluctuation of hormone levels. It would be worth trying an HRT patch since this provides steadier hormone levels and may well not worsen the migraines. If you are postmenopausal, period-free HRT may be less likely to trigger your migraines. However, the effect of HRT on migraines can be unpredictable!

I had a hysterectomy 6 years ago leaving my ovaries intact. In May this year I had to have my right ovary removed as a cyst was found on it. My left ovary was left intact to provide the hormones that I was told I still needed. Unfortunately, following some menopausal symptoms, I have been told that my remaining ovary is not functioning and I am going through an early menopause; I am only 42. I have been told that I will need to take HRT, and I am certainly not feeling too good at the moment because I am suffering quite badly with hot flushes and night sweats. I'm worried because I'm a migraine sufferer and concerned in case HRT makes them worse. I started migraines with aura when I became pregnant at 19 and was unable to take the contraceptive pill as it made them a lot worse. My migraines have become much less frequent now and I wonder if this is because of the drop in my hormones or just a natural improvement. I feel I am in a catch 22 situation. I know I should take HRT at my age.

I would agree that it would be worth trying HRT in view of your young age, but I appreciate your concerns in relation to the migraines. The association between migraines, menopause and HRT is complex – some women do find that migraines reduce with the onset of the menopause, some worsen. Some find an improvement with HRT, some worse! For some women, migraine is worsened by the fluctuating hormone levels and also possibly by the fluctuations that you get by taking a daily hormone tablet. Therefore, if you do decide to try HRT, I would suggest a patch or gel rather than a tablet and that you start with a low dose. If you find that the migraines do worsen with HRT, then other non-hormonal treatments can be used.

'Allergy' to HRT

Even though I am only 43, I have been on HRT for 5 years and for 4 of them I used patches. I am troubled with dizzy spells and 'thick' heads and sometimes feel that I am not in control. People told me that this was stress but it turned out that I was allergic to the patch and I am now on tablets. However, my weight increased by 2 stone and I lost my sex drive so I then changed to a different HRT prescription. Now I'm getting the same symptoms as before and I have reached the point where I don't want to continue with this course anymore. I have been advised against this because of the possibility of osteoporosis in later life, but I am now concerned that HRT is not for me and that the symptoms I experience will stay with me regardless. Please can you advise me of the best course of action?

If the HRT types do not suit you and you have not had a trial off HRT, then it would be worthwhile seeing how you feel on nothing. We often advise a trial off treatment to 'get back to baseline' since often, after a few years of changing from one type of HRT to another, you don't know whether or not the HRT is actually helping or causing problems. If on stopping HRT you feel better and decide to stay off treatment, then there might be a concern about your increased risk of osteoporosis in the future, but this can be monitored, perhaps by consideration of a bone density measurement around the age of 50. Other factors that can help your bones are a healthy diet, weight-bearing exercise and not smoking. There are lots of benefits of HRT but it does not suit everyone.

Weight gain

Will I put on weight if I take HRT?

Although many women appear to put on weight when they take HRT and often blame HRT for weight gain, many women put on weight around the time of the menopause anyway without taking HRT. Studies have shown that there is no difference in weight gain between women who take HRT and those that don't. Often, women who feel better when taking HRT are more motivated to eat healthily and exercise, so may in fact lose weight. However, some women do retain fluid when taking HRT, particularly in the first few months of treatment. If this doesn't settle after 3 months or so, therapy can be adjusted by reducing the dose, changing the type or changing the route. Women respond differently to different types and routes of both oestrogen and progestogen and sometimes several changes are required to find the type that suits best. A new type of HRT for post-menopausal women contains a progestogen that specifically reduces the fluid-retaining effect of oestrogen and may be helpful for some women.

RISKS OF HRT

Over the last few years there has been much publicity surrounding risks of HRT. This has followed the publication of some large, highly publicised trials. The first of these was the Women's Health Initiative (WHI) trial in America which initially reported in 2002 and further in 2004. This trial tested the effects of HRT compared with placebo in over 26,000 healthy, postmenopausal women aged 50–79 years. Those who had not had a hysterectomy (over 16,000) took either oestrogen combined with progestogen, or placebo (an inactive substance). Those who had had a hysterectomy (over 10,000) took either oestrogen or placebo. Risks of venous thrombosis (blood clot), breast cancer, heart attack and stroke following HRT were reported as alarming percentage increases, but in fact absolute risks were small.

The British Million Women study, reported in 2003, also showed an increased risk of breast cancer in users of HRT but the design of this study has been much criticised, and it has been stated that the risk has been overestimated. Nevertheless, we must be informed of risks of treatment, even if those risks are small, and we must try to balance risks against benefits.

Venous thrombosis

Studies have consistently demonstrated an increased risk of venous thrombosis (such as a blood clot in the leg) with the use of HRT. From the WHI trial mentioned above, venous thrombosis occurred in 3 per 1000 women aged 50–59 not taking HRT over 5 years, and in 8 per 1000 women aged 60–69. In women taking combined HRT for 5 years, there were an extra 4 cases per 1000 women aged 50–59 and an extra 9 per 1000 women aged 60–69. In women taking oestrogen only for 5 years, there was an extra 1 case per 1000 women aged 50–59 and an extra 4 per 1000 women aged 60–69. The greatest risk appears to be within the first year of use and is par-ticularly relevant to women who have other risk factors for thrombosis, including previous or family history of venous throm-boembolism, advancing age, obesity or underlying blood clotting problem. There is some evidence that non-tablet oestrogen, such as a patch, may not confer the same increased risk and can be considered in women at risk of thromboembolism but who need HRT. Also, lower doses of tablet oestrogen possibly carry a lower risk than the standard dose. Reassuringly, from further analysis of the WHI trial, for women of *normal* weight aged between 50 and 59, the rate of blood clot from HRT is 0.8 per 1000 women per year, which is in fact very similar to the rate with placebo.

I've been on HRT for a few years. I'm going to Australia for a holiday and am worried about getting a blood clot on the flight. Is this likely?

The main, albeit small risk of HRT causing a blood clot is within the first year of use. Therefore, if you've not had any problems by now, it is unlikely to cause problems. Long-haul flights may increase the risk because of the long periods of immobility. Therefore it is important to keep moving your feet and legs as much as possible and drink plenty of water or decaffeinated drinks, avoiding alcohol and coffee. Leg exercises are now usually shown in the in-flight magazines and can be carried out easily: these will include circular foot movements by rotating the ankles; pointing your toes away from the leg and then pulling your foot up towards the shin; and simply going for occasional walks up and down the plane during the flight. Try to avoid sitting with crossed legs or ankles. Some people advise taking a single small-dose aspirin before travelling to keep the blood thinner, but some people cannot take aspirin because of other medical problems. Flight stockings help to keep the circulation moving but you should check that they fit properly and are not too tight.

I know someone who developed a blood clot after surgery. I am taking HRT – do I need to stop my HRT before my knee operation?

Surgery can increase the risk of a blood clot but, if the operation is a minor procedure following which you will be mobile quite quickly, then there is no need to stop your HRT, as long as your surgeon knows what you are taking and can then offer anticlotting measures. If your surgery is major and is likely to be followed by a period of immobility, then HRT can be stopped beforehand. The increased risk of clotting disappears rapidly when HRT is stopped, so you could stop it just 4 weeks before planned surgery. Alternatively, it can be continued as recommended for minor surgery as long as anticlotting measures are taken.

Breast cancer

It has for some time been well accepted that long-term HRT use (over 5 years after the age of 50) confers a small increased risk of breast cancer, and the figures often quoted are those from Professor Valerie Beral's work (Table 8.5).

From both the WHI trial and Million Women study mentioned above, it appears that oestrogen-only HRT carries less risk than oestrogen combined with progestogen with respect to breast cancer and long-term use, the WHI trial in particular demonstrating no increased risk with oestrogen-only HRT taken for up to 7 years. In fact, the women who took oestrogen-only HRT had a reduced risk of breast cancer compared with those taking placebo. This reduction was not significant when all the women were grouped together, but was significant in those women who had not taken HRT before the trial. For those taking combined HRT, overall, it was initially reported that combined HRT probably accounts for three to four extra cases of breast cancer per 1000 women who take combined HRT from the age of 50 for 5 years. However, the final analysis of the trial showed

Table 8.5 RISK OF BREAST CANCER IN WOMEN TAKING HRT*

Years of taking HRT	Number of cases of breast cancer per 1000 women aged 50–70	Number of extra cases per 1000 women
0	45	0
over 5	47	2
over 10	51	6
over 15	57	12

* Figures produced by the Collaborative Group on Hormonal Factors in Breast Cancer (1997)

Breast cancer and HRT: collaborative reanalysis of data from 51 epidemiological studies of 52,705 women with breast cancer and 108,411 women without breast cancer. *Lancet* **350**: 1047–59.

that the increased risk of breast cancer applied only to those women who had taken combined HRT for more than 5 years **before** commencing the trial and then took the HRT for the 5 years of the trial. There was **no** increase in women in the trial taking HRT who had not taken it prior to the trial. The increased risk of breast cancer as shown by the WHI trial, therefore applies only to women who take combined HRT for more than 10 years after the age of 50. After stopping HRT for 5 years, the risk returns to baseline.

It has been shown that women who develop breast cancer while taking HRT have a lower mortality rate than those developing breast cancer when not taking HRT, possibly because HRT may lead to less aggressive tumours.

If HRT is commenced because of an early menopause after hysterectomy, it can be continued until the age of 50 years without concern about the increased risk of breast cancer. The risk of breast cancer from taking HRT from the time of an early menopause up to the age of 50 is thought to be similar to the risk for a woman who continued having a normal menstrual cycle up to the age of 50. However, it is thought that having an early surgical menopause and not taking HRT reduces the risk of breast cancer, but increases the risk of osteoporosis. Generally, following an early menopause from whatever reason, it is recommended that HRT is taken up to the age of 50. At around the age of 50, the decision as to whether or not to continue HRT should be made. This is the same decision that any woman becoming menopausal at the normal menopausal age would have to make, i.e. whether or not to commence HRT.

When you are considering the relationship between HRT and breast cancer, it is important to realise that there are other factors than the 5 years' use of HRT that may increase the risk of breast cancer as much, if not more. These include:

- more than 2–3 units of alcohol per day

- postmenopausal obesity

- a high intake of saturated fat

- having your first child after the age of 30 years, and

- having a natural menopause after the age of 54 years.

I've been on HRT for 15 years but am now trying to wean myself off and for the past 4 months I have taken nothing. However, the return of the hot flushes and other symptoms (tiredness, aching shoulders, irritable bladder), are debilitating. I am beginning to ask myself if the (presumed) risk of breast cancer is worth it. It is so difficult to weigh up some percentage risk reduction in the future with the discomfort I am currently undergoing. What is your opinion?

If your menopausal symptoms are affecting your quality of life and nothing else helps, then it is likely that the benefits of HRT out-weigh the risks. The risk of breast cancer with HRT has to be considered, but it is a small risk and control of your symptoms is important. There are many factors that influence a woman's perception of risk and her decision-making, such as the information to which she has access, the seriousness of the condition to which the risk relates, but most importantly, the presence and severity of menopausal symptoms. Women with severe symptoms can find them so debilitating that they are prepared to accept some risk.

Endometrial cancer

Oestrogen-only therapy given to women with an intact uterus (womb) increases the risk of endometrial hyperplasia (thickening) and cancer. Oestrogen combined with cyclical progestogen (sequential HRT) reduces this risk but does not eliminate it. Sequential HRT given for over 5 years does confer a small increased risk of endometrial cancer but no increased risk appears to apply to oestrogen combined with continuous progestogen (continuous combined or period-free therapy). Research is now looking at the possibility of using very low-dose oestrogen, which would still control menopausal symptoms but not stimulate the womb lining, avoiding the need for progestogen, but further trials are awaited.

I've had normal bleeds on my HRT previously but recently my bleeds have become heavier and last longer. Should I get this checked out or will it sort itself out?

Any change in the pattern of bleeding, such as the bleeds becoming heavier, irregular or longer on monthly bleed-type HRT, should be reported and investigated, since there might be some changes within the womb lining. Your doctor will probably refer you to your local hospital and investigation is simple. The type of investigation depends on what facilities are available locally. It may be in the form of an ultrasound scan to look at the womb to see if you have fibroids, or may involve having a sample taken from the womb lining (by passing a small plastic tube into the womb through the cervix). You may have a procedure called a hysteroscopy, which involves looking into the womb with a telescope. This can either be done in the outpatient clinic with some local anaesthetic, or if necessary under general anaesthetic.

Ovarian cancer

Some studies have suggested a possible link between long-term HRT use (oestrogen only) and a small increased risk of ovarian cancer but this has not been confirmed.

RISK OR BENEfiT?

Heart disease

For many years, HRT was thought to be protective against heart problems (cardioprotective) with observational studies (where women are simply followed up and doctors observe whether or not they take HRT and whether they subsequently develop any disease, rather than randomly being allocated to taking HRT or not) showing reduced risks of heart attack and stroke in users of HRT. However, the initial reports from the WHI trial showed early, though transient, small increased risks in heart disease. Later analysis showed that women who were fewer than 10 years postmenopausal when starting combined HRT and those women who had undergone hysterectomy taking oestrogen only, showed **no** increased risk of heart attack during the trial. Final analysis of the increase with combined HRT in women who started HRT more than 10 years after the menopause, demonstrated the increase to be in the first year of the trial, with a decrease in events thereafter and **no** overall increase in heart disease by the end of the trial. Further, the oestrogen only part of the trial showed a **reduction** in those taking oestrogen, which was most apparent in women aged 50 to 59 years.

Recent information from the Nurses' Health Study has shown that women who commenced HRT near the time of the menopause in fact had a **reduced** risk of heart disease compared with similar women not taking HRT.

It is possible that the dose, type and route of HRT used are important in this type of risk, as is the timing of commencement of therapy. It is very likely that use of both oestrogen-only and combined HRT started early in the menopause has no harmful effects on the risk of heart disease but that, once disease of the arteries has developed, commencing HRT may promote further damage. It is therefore very unlikely that HRT given to women in the early menopause for control of menopausal symptoms will be harmful for the heart, and may still yet be proven without doubt to be beneficial if started early enough.

Stroke

The change has hit me really badly and I need some treatment but I'm terrified of taking HRT because my friend told me it might cause a stroke.

Both oestrogen-only and combined HRT were shown to be associated with a small increased risk of stroke in the WHI trial. In women aged 50–59 not taking HRT, a stroke owing to narrowing of the blood vessels to the brain occurred in 3 per 1000 women over a period of 5 years; 5 years of HRT therapy was associated with 1 additional case. Therefore if you have no other risk factors, the risk of stroke from HRT is extremely small and, in fact, there is some evidence that lower doses of oestrogen than were used in the WHI trial can reduce the risk of stroke compared with placebo. A more recent study from Sweden showed no association between the use of HRT and stroke.

Alzheimer's disease

Debate also surrounds the role of HRT in the development of Alzheimer's disease, some studies showing a reduction in risk in HRT users but the WHI showing an increased risk, although this was only in women who were aged over 75 years. A major difference between trials such as the WHI, initially reporting increased risks of dementia and heart disease with HRT, and the observational studies which have often shown a reduced risk of such problems with HRT, is that, in the WHI trial, women started HRT some time after the menopause (only 10% were in the early menopausal years and, on average, the women were 12 years postmenopausal), whereas in observational studies, HRT has generally been started early in the menopausal years to control menopausal symptoms. It has been proposed that there is a 'window of opportunity' whereby, if HRT is started early enough, it may be beneficial not only for control of symptoms and prevention of osteoporosis, but also for prevention of heart disease and dementia.

However, HRT should not currently be used primarily to prevent heart disease, stroke or Alzheimer's disease. The debate continues.

CONTRAINDICATIONS FOR HRT

Are there any circumstances when HRT should not be used?

The list below gives some circumstances when it is usually inappropriate to take HRT:

- pregnancy
- undiagnosed abnormal vaginal bleeding (this should be investigated before commencing HRT)
- active recent blood clot (thrombosis) or heart attack (myocardial infarction)
- suspected or active breast or endometrial (womb) cancer
- active liver disease with abnormal liver function tests
- porphyria (an inherited condition caused by disturbance in the metabolism of porphyrin pigments)
- history of inherited clotting disorders, e.g. factor V Leiden.

In some of these situations, HRT may be prescribed, but only after discussion with a specialist.

9 | Non-HRT drug therapies

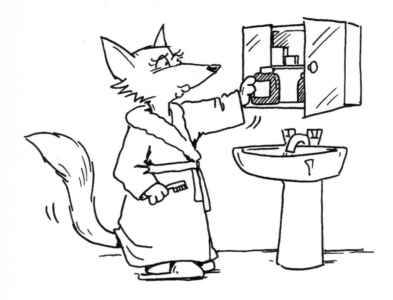

Several non-HRT drugs are used for menopausal symptoms, though it should be noted that HRT and clonidine are currently the only preparations that are licensed for menopausal flushes.

ALTERNATIVES FOR flUSHES

Clonidine (Dixarit)

This drug is used for migraine or high blood pressure and has been shown to reduce hot flushes compared with placebo to a modest degree. It is often used as a treatment for flushes in a dose ranging from two to three 25 mcg tablets twice a day – the dose is adjusted according to response. It is usually well tolerated but side effects include difficulty sleeping, dry mouth, dizziness, constipation and sedation. Tell your doctor if you are taking antihypertensives also as these can interact with clonidine.

I'm taking clonidine for the night sweats . . . well I only had four sweats last night, so I am keeping my fingers crossed because the tablets seem to be helping so far. The only side effects I have had are a dry mouth and a slight headache, but I can put up with that. How long should I take the clonidine for?

As for any therapy taken for night sweats or flushes, it is worth having a trial off treatment every couple of years or so to see if the symptoms are still present and therefore if treatment is still required. We are not aware of any long-term problems with the use of clonidine.

I was on clonidine in the past with good results, but the flushes came back after I stopped taking it. I have now been put back on clonidine but am waiting for it to kick back in. My only problem is that this time it is making me so sleepy – I actually fell asleep at my computer the other day – not a good move as I am in a new job! I notice that my skin is wrinkling rapidly too. What can I do about the sleepiness and is the wrinkly skin due to the clonidine?

Feeling sleepy has been noted as a side effect. If you are on a high dose, e.g. three tablets twice daily, then cutting down the dose may reduce the sleepiness while still helping your flushes. If this doesn't help and the sleepiness is really bad, then you may want to try something else. It is very unlikely that the clonidine is causing your skin to wrinkle more rapidly. This is a common problem that may be related to the lack of oestrogen with the onset of the menopause, but sadly age has an effect also! A good quality skin moisturiser should help.

Progestogens

Medroxyprogesterone acetate (MPA, Provera), megestrol acetate (Megace) and norethisterone (Primolut) are synthetic forms of progesterone, which can sometimes reduce hot flushes and sweats. They may also offer a degree of bone protection. They are most often prescribed to women who cannot take oestrogen, for example after breast cancer treatment. However, with recent studies suggesting that progestogens may be more influential in increasing the risk of breast cancer than oestrogen alone, uncertainty currently exists regarding the use of progestogen after breast cancer. The side effects of these drugs can sometimes outweigh the benefits – weight gain and bloating being common. There may also be an increased risk of clotting with higher doses of progestogens.

> *By accident, I found that a drug called norethisterone stopped my flushes completely. The drug was prescribed to stop my periods (which were very troublesome at the time) during the month that I got married and I realised later that I no longer suffered from the hot flushes or sweats. I have taken it on a very low dosage ever since with my doctor's blessing and avoided the flush symptoms altogether. I have tried stopping the drug for a week to see what happens and they come back – I go back on the drug and they stop again. How does it stop periods and how long should I stay on it for?*

Norethisterone is a synthetic progesterone. The lining of the womb is shed (because of menstruation) when the progesterone level falls after the lining has been stimulated by oestrogen – this happens in the natural monthly cycle. By taking this progestogen and preventing the fall in level, the lining does not shed. Perhaps after another year or so, it would be reasonable to stop again to see what your own cycle is like and to see if it is still needed.

SSRI drugs (selective serotonin reuptake inhibitors)

The belief that a variety of chemical reactions involving serotonin, noradrenaline and dopamine are instrumental in the initiation of a flush has led to trials of drugs that affect the levels of serotonin and noradrenaline. SSRIs are a class of antidepressant drugs whose actions include an effect on the 'thermostat' receptor as well as helping depression.

I have been struggling to find a treatment to help my flushes and mood swings. I tried several types of HRT but whatever I tried just didn't seem to suit me. My doctor has now suggested trying an antidepressant. I really don't think I'm depressed – although I do feel a bit down about it all. I'm sure it's just the awful flushes and my not sleeping that's causing all the problems. How can an antidepressant help?

The antidepressants known as SSRIs have also been shown to reduce flushes, not by their antidepressant effect but by their action on the chemical serotonin. Serotonin appears to play a part in the function of the 'thermostat', which is located in the brain and regulates temperature. The doses of these drugs that are used for menopausal flushes are usually much lower than those used for depression.

They have been studied and widely used effectively for reducing flushes in women surviving breast cancer. Examples are venlafaxine (Efexor), fluoxetine (Prozac) and paroxetine (Seroxat).

Venlafaxine has an effect on both serotonin and noradrenaline and, when women were given doses of 37.5 mg, 75 mg and 150 mg daily, their flushes were reduced by 37, 61 and 61% respectively, compared with women given a placebo treatment who had a reduction of 27%. The usual starting dose is 37.5 mg daily with gradual increase in dose if necessary to reduce the risk of side effects, which include nausea, dry mouth, dizziness, problems with sleeping, agitation and confusion. In 2004, the CSM (Committee on Safety of

Medicines) advised doctors to be cautious in prescribing venlafaxine because of concerns about a toxic effect on the heart, and also toxicity if an overdose were to be taken. It was recommended that treatment with venlafaxine should be initiated only by specialist mental health practitioners and that it should not be used by people who have heart disease, high blood pressure or an imbalance of certain substances such as potassium in their blood. However, after further investigation, these restrictions have now been lifted and venlafaxine can still be prescribed in low doses for menopausal hot flushes.

Paroxetene, 12.5–25 mg daily, produces a 50% reduction in flushes; fluoxetene, 20 mg daily, produces a 60% reduction. Interactions have been reported with drugs that act on the central nervous system, and warfarin. The dose of SSRIs can be started low and increased gradually to minimise any side effects. Hot flushes are reduced further after higher-dose SSRIs but the side effects are worse.

Gabapentin

Gabapentin (Neurontin), a drug used to treat epilepsy, migraine and nerve-related pain, has been shown to reduce flushes by about 45%. It may be particularly beneficial for the symptoms of aches, pains and tingling sensations, which many menopausal women suffer. Possible side effects include dizziness, fatigue, tremor and weight gain but these can be reduced by increasing the dose gradually.

It should be noted that neither SSRI drugs nor gabapentin are licensed to be used for menopausal symptoms. Although studies have shown beneficial effects, they have often been small studies and of short duration. These drugs would be recommended by a specialist rather than by your general practitioner.

ALTERNATIVES FOR VAGINAL AND BLADDER SYMPTOMS

Many women suffer from symptoms owing to thinning of the tissues of the vagina and bladder. Sadly, these symptoms are hugely under-reported and very much undertreated, often because of embarrassment and lack of awareness of the availability of effective treatments. Symptoms include vaginal dryness, irritation, discharge, discomfort during intercourse, and passing urine frequently and with discomfort.

Vaginal oestrogen can be very effective and should not be regarded in the same way as systemic oestrogen with respect to possible side effects and risks, since the drug is concentrated in the vaginal and bladder tissues with minimal risk of absorption into the body itself.

For women who prefer non-hormonal treatments, some effective preparations are available such as Replens, a moisturising gel that contains purified water (78.8%) as the active ingredient. This clings to the vaginal walls and is slowly released for up to 3 days until the cells are shed naturally. During this time, one application of Replens delivers continuous moisturisation to thin cells, while increasing blood flow to the vaginal walls and balancing acidity for a healthy vaginal environment. It offers a hormone-free solution for the treatment of vaginal atrophy (thinning) and dryness, itching, irritation, discomfort or pain during intercourse. Replens is available over the counter and ReplensMD is available on prescription.

Also available is Sylk, a natural lubricant made from an extract of the kiwi fruit vine, which appears to help vaginal dryness. Other lubricants such as KY Jelly and Senselle can be used at the time of intercourse itself.

I have cystitis and wonder what might help?

Straightforward cystitis is usually treated with antibiotics and increased fluid intake but urinary problems owing to the menopause may mimic cystitis. Urinary problems, such as passing urine very often and incontinence, may require specific assessment and treatments aimed directly at helping your bladder function and support. You can read more about pelvic floor exercises in Chapter 7. Women are often too embarrassed to report bladder problems, particularly poor control and hence leakage but effective treatments are available. Drugs such as tolterodine (Detrusitol) and solifenacin succinate (Vesicare) can reduce the frequency and urgency of passing urine, while duloxetine (Yentreve) specifically aims to reduce stress incontinence. If measures such as pelvic floor exercises, bladder retraining and drugs are ineffective, then an operation can be considered. Recent advances have led to the development of operations that are quick, require only a short time in hospital and are very successful.

There is a question about cranberry juice for cystitis in Chapter 10.

OSTEOPOROSIS

Non-HRT options for osteoporosis are discussed in Chapters 4 and 10.

10 | Alternative and complementary therapies

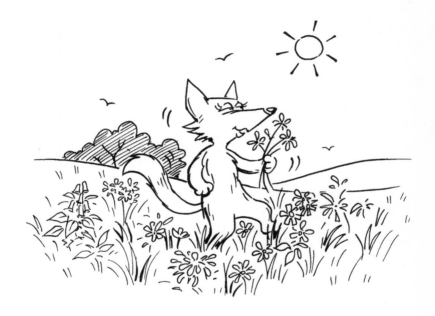

Over the last few years, there has been increasing interest in, and use of, 'over-the-counter' alternative therapies for treating menopausal symptoms, particularly since HRT has been receiving extensive adverse publicity; 'natural' alternatives are regarded as 'safe' by the general public. (There is also interest in prescribed alternatives to HRT and these are discussed in Chapter 9.) Dietary supplements and over-the-counter alternative therapies are often used and one report found that 42% of adults had used some form of alternative therapy, yet very few users inform their doctors that they are taking such therapies. This is of concern since some products can interact with other medications. Therefore it is very important to tell your doctor if you are taking alternative therapies while on prescribed medicine.

Some alternative preparations have shown encouraging effects in reducing menopausal symptoms, improving lipid levels (blood fats) and protecting bone, but many commercial preparations vary hugely in the actual content of active ingredients, have not been subject to rigorous scientific investigation for effect, and have no long-term safety information. The plants' active chemicals can also vary, depending on their genetics, harvesting time, processing and individual metabolisms.

If you are using alternative therapies, it can be very difficult to know which one to try and often it is a case of trial and error – take care to try only one product at a time.

SUPPLEMENTS

Phytoestrogens

The interest in phytoestrogens has developed not least because of the epidemiological evidence that women in areas of the world such as Japan and other parts of Asia who consume diets rich in these compounds appear to have much lower incidences of 'western diseases' such as heart disease, osteoporosis, and cancers of the breast, colon and womb. Women in these countries do not appear to experience hot flushes and sweats as much as women do in the western world, although the difference may also be related to other factors such as cultural differences in their attitude to the menopause.

Phytoestrogens are a group of naturally occurring compounds derived from plants that have oestrogenic activity or are metabolised into compounds that have oestrogenic activity. They were first identified in the early 1930s, have a similar chemical structure to oestrogen and bind to the oestrogen receptors. They bind most strongly to those oestrogen receptors found in bone, bowel, lung and blood vessels, rather than to the receptors found in the breast and uterus (womb). As a group of compounds they exhibit many properties, such as anti-inflammatory effects, and can boost oestrogen effects, even though the dose is very small.

Phytoestrogens have been shown in some clinical trials to reduce hot flushes significantly, although many of the trials were undertaken over short periods, e.g. only 3 months. Some trials have shown limited effect and little benefit compared with a placebo (a non-active treatment). Limited research has so far shown a weak to modest beneficial effect on the cardiovascular system, possible beneficial effect on bone, suggestion of a protective effect on breast cancer, colon cancer and lung cancer, and little effect on improving vaginal symptoms. It appears that life-time use of phytoestrogens may be required to provide the protective effects. Regarding adverse effects, only one study has shown that phytoestrogens can stimulate the

---

Box 10.1 DIETARY SOURCES OF PHYTOESTROGENS
OR PLANT OESTROGENS

- **Cereals**: oats, barley, rye, brown rice, couscous and bulgar wheat

- **Seeds**: sunflower, sesame, pumpkin, poppy, linseeds*

- **Pulses**: soybeans and all soy-based products*

- **Beans**: chickpeas, kidney beans, haricot beans, broad beans, green split peas, lentils

- **Vegetables**: red onions, green beans, celery, sweet peppers, sage, garlic, broccoli, tomatoes and bean sprouts

- **Commercial products** are also available, such as Bergen bread, Provamel yoghurts and 'So Good' milk

  * Soya and linseeds are the richest sources.

womb lining, causing an unwanted thickening, but in this study very high doses were used.

Phytoestrogens can be taken either by increasing dietary intake or in the form of supplements. They are found in about 300 plants, particularly legumes such as peas and beans. To rely on dietary intake alone would involve the ingestion of large amounts of legumes – probably too large to be practical. (See Table 10.1)

There are four subclasses of phytoestrogens that have been most investigated: isoflavones, flavones, lignans and coumestrans. They occur naturally in an inactive form but are converted by intestinal bacteria to biologically active products, which can be absorbed into the bloodstream. Isoflavones are the most common form of phyto-estrogens and include genistein, daidzein and glycitin. In Japan, the average intake of isoflavones is 50 mg per day compared with 5 mg per day in the western world. A dietary intake of at least 40 mg per day is thought to be required to have beneficial effect.

I read that eating more soya will help my flushes. How does it work and what can I buy that has soya in it?

Soybeans are a good source of phytoestrogens, namely isoflavones, which are concentrated just below the seed leaves and in the first layer of leaves. Isoflavones from plant sources need to be broken down in the bowel by bowel bacteria before they can become active. The huge variation between people for absorption rate and presence of bowel bacteria means that there is a concomitant huge variation in how effective these sources will be; there is thought to be up to a 10-fold variation in the amount of phytoestrogen that becomes available because of differing metabolisms between individuals. When broken down, the compounds have both oestrogenic and anti-oestro-genic activity. The oestrogenic effect should help reduce hot flushes but research has shown varying results. Foods derived from soybeans include soya milk, tofu, miso (a Japanese product), soy sauce and soy protein concentrate, which is an ingredient in many foods.

I gather that phytoestrogens are good for the menopause.
I don't really want to change my diet, which I think is quite
healthy, so can I buy a phytoestrogen supplement?

Many supplements are now available that provide varying amounts and types of phytoestrogens. Red clover is an excellent source of the phytoestrogen isoflavones, and an example is Novogen Redclover (Novogen). Red clover, marketed for instance as Promensil in the USA, has been endorsed by the Food and Drug Administration as a cholesterol-lowering and prostate cancer-reducing product. Promensil is an extract of red clover and contains the isoflavones daidzein, genistein, biochanin (which is broken down to genistein) and formononetin (which is broken down to daidzein). Promensil contains 40 mg of isoflavones per tablet and the recommended dose is 1 tablet per day.

Other phytoestrogen supplements currently available include Estroven (soy-based), Nutrafem (a dual formulation of extracts made from green bean phytoestrogens), Menopace (a formulation of 21 nutrients including soy isoflavones, vitamins, minerals and co-factors) and Tofupill. Tofupill is derived from a variety of soybean that is high in phytoestrogen content and is made by a process that retains the whole group of phytoestrogen compounds. Recommended dose is 1 capsule twice daily.

I had breast cancer a few years ago and am now having
flushes. My doctor told me that I can't take HRT but I was
wondering if I could take a natural oestrogen supplement?

Because of lack of research on the effect of natural oestrogens, or phytoestrogens, after breast cancer, such products should currently be used with caution. Some breast surgeons and oncologists believe that even the tiny amounts of oestrogen can have an adverse effect, but opinion is currently divided. It would be worth having a talk with your doctor or a specialist in menopausal matters at a local health clinic.

I recently started taking a red clover supplement – it has helped my mood swings and the hot flushes. I read up on it on the internet and decided to give it a try. I am surprised that I got a proper period 3 weeks into taking it and I am trying to find out if this is to be expected.

Red clover should not stimulate the womb lining and therefore should not cause bleeding. The bleed may have been unrelated to the red clover and a coincidence. If this is the first bleed for a year or more, then you should see your doctor to have this checked out.

Black cohosh

Actaea (formerly *Cimicifuga*) *racemosa*, commonly known as bugbane, is a member of the buttercup family and a woodland perennial. It was used by the North American Indians who called it 'black snakeroot' because of its gnarled black root, which contains a complex mixture of natural chemicals. They boiled up the root and drank the tea, which was used to ease menstrual cramps and childbirth pains. Black cohosh is one of the most widely studied botanicals for menopausal symptoms. It was thought that it had similar properties to plant oestrogens and binds to the same receptors in the body that oestrogen does, although recent research has suggested that it does not act like an oestrogen but that it acts on serotonin receptors (see Chapter 9), relieving hot flushes and mood through a serotonin effect. It may help with the mood swings, depression and weepiness that can be associated with hormone fluctuation. Placebo-controlled trials have shown that black cohosh can reduce flushes in doses ranging from 39 to 127 mg of a standardised extract (Remifemin) daily, the higher doses having a greater effect; but not all studies have shown this. It does not appear to have any effect on bone, the cardiovascular system, breasts or endometrium. Studies have generally been of short duration and therefore little information is available for long-term effect.

It is available as a 'tincture' by putting drops into water to drink, and also as tablets. The doses vary with the product. The product marketed as Remifemin contains 40 mg and is taken as 1 tablet per day. There have been reports of liver damage such as hepatitis in some women while taking black cohosh but, since there have been very few cases out of many, many women using black cohosh, it has a very good safety profile. It probably should not be used if you have a history of liver problems and should be used with caution if you have high blood pressure.

I'm interested in trying a natural alternative to HRT and have heard that black cohosh is good, but I'm very confused by what is available – lots of products contain a whole mixture of things along with black cohosh and others just black cohosh. My husband and I stand in Holland & Barrett for ages looking at all the various products and we are as confused as each other! Which is best?

Many products are available despite the lack of scientific evidence on their effect. Because there has been some research carried out on black cohosh that found that there may be a beneficial effect on menopausal symptoms, then it probably should be taken on its own, rather than in a mixture, if you want to try it. Mixtures only increase the danger of interactions.

Agnus castus

This is a compound known as 'monks' pepper' or 'chasteberry extract'. The fruit of this plant has long been thought to influence sex hormones, modifying the balance between oestrogen and progesterone. *Agnus castus* has been fairly well studied and is available as a tincture or in tablet form. The tablets have a very strong smell and most people find the tincture easier to take. It is often found in combination with black cohosh and other herbs. Studies have demonstrated value for the treatment of premenstrual tension/syndrome (PMS). It may be useful for menstrual irregularity in the perimenopausal phase when hormones are fluctuating wildly. Very little is known about its effect on other menopausal symptoms. *Agnus castus* is useful only if hormones are not already being taken. It has been used widely in Germany where herbal medicines are often used alongside traditional medicines, for impaired ovarian function, period problems and PMS.

Evening primrose oil

This oil is well known for its breast pain-relieving properties. Evening primrose oil is derived from the seeds of *Oenothera biennis* (evening primrose) and was available as Efamast or Epogam on prescription for breast pain and eczema respectively. These have now been withdrawn as prescription drugs but they can be bought over the counter, either as evening primrose oil or borage oil. There are a variety of strengths and potencies. Look for the amount of GLA (gamma linoleic acid) in each capsule. Aim for 240 mg per day for at least 2 months and then try reducing the dose. It might be useful for breast pain, but is unlikely to be helpful for hot flushes. The best studies do not show such an effect. Adverse effects include headache, diarrhoea and nausea.

Ginkgo biloba

Ginkgo biloba is known as the maidenhair tree or the 'memory tree'. Extracts are reported to be helpful with circulation, and therefore memory, by helping improve glucose and oxygen supply to the brain, controlled trials demonstrating improved brain function and memory. It may rarely increase the risk of bleeding by affecting the blood clotting system and so it is best not to take it with drugs that reduce clotting, such as warfarin, aspirin or the coumarins.

Dong quai

Dong quai has been used for many years as a Chinese medicine. It is derived from the root of *Angelica sinensis*, a perennial plant found in southwest China, and is often found in combination products. There has been debate as to whether or not it has oestrogenic activity; studies so far suggest not. No evidence exists to demonstrate a beneficial effect on menopausal symptoms compared with placebo and there have been occasional reports of bleeding when it is taken along with warfarin.

Ginseng (*Panax ginseng*)

This is a herb found in China and Korea. Limited research has shown no benefit on hot flushes compared with placebo, although there was improvement in depression and general wellbeing. There have been case reports of postmenopausal bleeding and breast tenderness with ginseng and possible interactions with warfarin and alcohol.

Femal

This is a herbal remedy made from pollen extracts and has been shown to be 20–30% better than placebo in a controlled trial to reduce menopausal symptoms. The main effect was on hot flushes after 2–3 months' treatment but there was also an improvement in tiredness, mood swings, dizziness, libido and general mood. There was no change in vaginal dryness, bleeding or hormone levels, suggesting that it does not have an oestrogenic action. However, its mechanism of action remains unclear. The recently reported trial showed promising results but it is accepted that the trial was fairly short and that larger trials are needed.

Kava kava (*Piper methysticum*)

This was first described by Captain Cook who was offered this as a 'welcome drink' when he arrived on the Polynesian islands. It was sold as being helpful in alleviating anxiety without being addictive, but it has now been withdrawn because of reported liver damage as a side effect.

Sage

This herb can be taken as a tea or as an extract. It may help meno-pausal symptoms by directly reducing the production of sweat but little scientific information is available. Take sage with caution if you have high blood pressure.

I was suffering very badly from hot flushes during the summer and made infusions from sage in a friend's garden. I let it cool down and just sipped it during the day and when I felt a flush coming on. It seemed to work. In fact, the flushes stopped completely within a week and they haven't recurred. But would they have stopped anyway? I wonder if the fact that I was away from work for a few weeks and stress free may have helped too.

There is no doubt that many factors interact to influence whether or not flushes occur and how bad they are, so it may well have been the stress-free environment that helped, rather than the sage. We do not have enough information from trials to know for sure if sage, and indeed many of the other alternative therapies, are effective. Many women may find a benefit but we don't know if they would have felt better anyway without any treatment. Sage seems to be available in many different forms – tablets, tincture, on its own, with other herbs and minerals, and you can get sage tea in different preparation forms in health food shops.

When my hot flushes and night sweats started over 2 years ago, I took a tincture of sage called Menosan and this did stop the flushes and sweats but only for a few weeks. Then they came back as strong and frequent as ever. Does this always happen?

Flushes often come and go and vary in severity. If the sage did help, it is very unlikely that it would then have caused symptoms to worsen.

St John's wort (*Hypericum perforatum*)

St John's wort is a wild flowering herb with distinctive yellow blooms. The extract, which is very popular in North America, acts by interacting with chemicals in the brain to have an antidepressant effect, possibly helping with the uptake of serotonin, a chemical vital for a feeling of wellbeing. It has been shown in some studies to be as effective as some traditional antidepressants but better tolerated without the side effects. It may be useful in women suffering mild to moderate anxiety and depressive symptoms at the menopause. Since several drug interactions may occur, **it should be used with caution if you are also taking: digoxin, the oral contraceptive pill, migraine drugs, anti-asthma drugs (theophylline), antiepileptic drugs, warfarin, cyclosporin and HIV drugs.** Always check with your doctor or pharmacist if you are taking other drugs and are considering using St John's wort. **It should not be taken along with any other antidepressant drugs.** It can also cause photosensitivity; a rash that develops in sunlight.

Maca

I have read about Maca and the results seem wonderful. What is it?

Maca is a root from Peru which looks like a little turnip or radish. Its Latin name is *Lepidium peruvianum chacon.* Maca contains high amounts of vitamins, minerals, enzymes and essential amino acids. It is said to enhance hormone production and is promoted as a libido enhancing agent, but very little scientific information on its effect is available.

Wild yam

Many HRT preparations are extracted from yams using a chemical conversion process. Wild yam progesterone creams have been widely promoted for hot flushes. However, the human body is incapable of breaking down the yam cream into progesterone; the chemical conversion cannot be duplicated in the body. The few available studies on the use of wild yam cream found no difference in menopausal symptoms compared with placebo.

Cranberry juice

Is it true that cranberry juice is good for cystitis and what else helps?

Women often become more prone to cystitis around the time of the menopause, or have symptoms that resemble cystitis. Simple things that may help include drinking plenty of water and liquids, such as cranberry juice, which help to keep the urine alkaline. Cranberry juice should not be taken if you are also taking warfarin since interactions may occur. Avoid lots of caffeine-containing drinks as they can aggravate bladder symptoms. Try not to get into the habit of going to the toilet often, 'just in case' – just go when you really need to but don't wait more than 4 hours during the day.

PROGESTERONE CREAM

'Natural' progesterone cream is available on a private prescription and is available in varying strengths. Two recent studies produced conflicting results on effects on hot flushes and sweats, one showing a small reduction and the other showing no change. When systemic oestrogen is used in women who have a uterus (womb) they must also take progestogen to protect the womb from cancer. **Natural progesterone is not suitable for giving protection to the womb** because of its lack of effect. There are claims that it can offer bone protection but these have not been confirmed. Therefore any individual at risk of osteoporosis should **not** consider this as an effective method for offering bone protection.

I read in a book that doctors have been getting it wrong for many years and that it's not oestrogen deficiency that causes menopausal problems but progesterone deficiency. Therefore we shouldn't be poisoning our bodies with oestrogen but should use natural progesterone cream. Is this true?

There has been a lot of publicity about the theory of the importance of progesterone deficiency and promotion of the use of progesterone cream. The studies used to 'prove' the theory have often been very old studies and what little scientific evidence there is has shown very little, if any, beneficial effects of progesterone cream. Masses of well-designed trials have demonstrated effects of oestrogen on menopausal problems and so, although it is accepted that there is still much to learn, it is strongly believed that it is actually oestrogen deficiency that plays the major role in the development of menopausal problems.

I started using progesterone cream 2 weeks ago and find it OK. I'm having days where I have hardly any flushes and days where I have a few every hour. I have ordered some black cohosh. Should I stop the cream as soon as I start taking black cohosh or take the two for a while?

The use of progesterone cream is controversial but, if you have found an improvement, then you probably don't need to start something else as well. However, if after a few more weeks there's not much benefit, then by all means try something else instead.

BIOIDENTICAL HORMONES

I saw an advert for bioidentical hormones, which sounded wonderful. What are they and are they really any good?

Bioidentical or bioequivalent hormones are synthetically engineered hormones that should be replicas of natural hormones but are made up in pharmacies and are not subject to the rigorous standards required by hormones sold by pharmaceutical companies. The hormones are often sold as combinations and evaluation of effect and safety is often lacking. Tests of salivary hormone levels may be offered in order to formulate a hormone combination likely to be beneficial to individuals but salivary hormone levels fluctuate widely and should not be relied upon.

DEHYDROEPIANDROSTERONE (DHEA)

Over recent years, there has been much interest in the use of DHEA for 'anti-ageing' therapy. It is a hormone produced by the adrenal gland and its production falls with age, with a 70–80% reduction starting in the 40s and reaching a maximum reduction after the age of 70, so that, by the age of 80, levels have declined to about 10% of those seen in early adulthood. DHEA is metabolised to oestrogen, progesterone and androstenedione. It is widely available in America as a food supplement and is used in the belief that it provides anti-ageing benefits. In the UK it is not readily available on prescription or in pharmacies but is increasingly purchased via the internet. Studies have been limited and, although it appears to improve libido, mood and wellbeing, it has not been shown to have any beneficial effect on hot flushes and sweats and its effect on bone and cardiovascular system is uncertain. Because of the lack of large trials, firm conclusions on the effect and long-term safety of DHEA cannot be made.

RISKS

I do feel sometimes that the medical profession does not treat menopausal symptoms seriously. Generally they advise against long-term use of HRT but offer little or nothing as a 'conventional medicine' alternative. So we are driven to ingesting all kinds of 'untested' herbal substances in a desperate search for symptomatic relief. Why aren't we given more specific information on herbal products?

The interest and expertise in treating menopausal symptoms does vary hugely between medical professionals and often conflicting advice is given. Over the last few years, the advice regarding HRT use has swung towards using it for the shortest duration necessary; however, in practice, since symptoms can continue in some women for a long time, the HRT can be continued for as long as it is thought to be beneficial and as long as there is an understanding of possible risks. Herbal products and other 'alternative' therapies are not subject to the same rigorous testing as drugs before they can be marketed, so useful scientific information on their effectiveness and safety profile is lacking. Therefore health professionals may not have any more information about them than yourself!

Lack of evidence does not necessarily mean that they don't work, but it does mean that we can't say that a particular product has been proven to help.

Many commercial products are available and new ones appear frequently. Although there is increasing evidence that some herbal and other preparations may be helpful, not only in reducing menopausal symptoms but also in preventing some diseases, there is a great need for further research into the effectiveness and safety of these products, both taken alone or in combination.

I hate the idea of putting strange things in my system unless it is absolutely necessary. I just wondered how many were taking nothing for the menopause and just changing their behaviour and eating habits instead, to see if that was helping them? Am I the only one who hates taking pills! Is it OK to turn down your doctor when he/she wants you to take medicines for the menopause (assuming it is not blood pressure or thyroid or something else that needs medicines to be treated)? It seems like a lot of women have been advised by their doctor to try HRT, or if not HRT, then phytoestrogens or something similar. I am really confused as to what I should be taking!

Adjusting diet and lifestyle is hugely important and often is all that's required. Unfortunately, many busy people find it easier to take a tablet than change their lifestyle since lifestyle changes need motivation and commitment. The menopause does not have to be treated with medicines, but for some women medicines can be very helpful. Any decision on how to manage your menopause should be made by you after gathering information and often after a full discussion with your doctor or practice nurse.

TECHNIQUES

There is very little scientific evidence that complementary therapies improve menopausal symptoms, yet many women who use such techniques report beneficial effects. Any therapy that allows you valuable 'timeout' is an investment in yourself and will help you cope with the menopause better.

Homeopathy

Homeopathy has been used for over 150 years and consists of the use of minute doses of a medicine that has matching characteristics to your symptoms, to stimulate the healing processes and reduce or eliminate the symptoms and the disorder. Exactly how it works is unclear. Homeopathic remedies are animal, plant or mineral in origin and are used in a highly diluted form. Some studies have shown a beneficial effect on menopausal symptoms, but the numbers of women in the studies were small and, when compared with placebo, there was no statistically significant difference. Side effects of homeopathy can occur and they include an initial and usually short-lived worsening of the symptoms that are being treated. This usually occurs within 10 days of taking the medicine. Generally, homeopathic treatments for menopausal symptoms appear to be well tolerated, safe and helpful for some women, but further trials will be required to determine their full effect. If you choose the homeopathic route, be sure to consult a trained homeopath (see Appendix 1). There may be a GP in your area who has been trained in this specialty. Some of the preparations commonly used are: *Aconitum*, *Lycopodium*, *Natrum muriaticum*, *Nux vomica*, *Pulsatilla*, *Sepia*, *Sulphur*, *Belladonna*, *Bryonia* and *Argentum*.

Alexander technique

This technique, developed by an Australian actor, is a method of adopting the ultimate posture to allow good breathing technique and help energy flow. There is a strong belief that many of us get into the habit of adopting poor posture, which causes unnecessary tension in muscles, leading to pain. Re-learning good posture and breathing technique is taught by Alexander teachers. Although there is no evidence of the effect of the Alexander technique specifically on the menopause, the breathing technique of paced respiration has been shown to reduce flushes by 39%.

Yoga

Yoga is often viewed as involving complex, physically challenging positions, but in fact the movements can be simple and easily achievable by most. The three principles of yoga are: breathing, postures and meditation. Yoga aims to relax muscles, improve suppleness, fitness and physical function, relax the mind and control stress. It should be practised regularly to be effective. Specific effects on menopausal symptoms are unknown but many women do find yoga beneficial.

Aromatherapy

Aromatherapy uses essential oils, which are extracted from plants and mainly applied to the skin. The combination of massage, smell and specific effect of the oils may help you to relax and relieve stress. Since stress is known to exacerbate menopausal symptoms, anything that reduces stress is likely to help. Essential oils used for menopausal problems include bergamot, cypress, clary sage, fennel, geranium and lavender.

Acupuncture

Acupuncture originates from traditional Chinese medicine and is now widely used in managing pain. Acupuncture aims to restore the balance of life energy, *qi*, which is said to be concentrated along channels within the body. These invisible channels have acupuncture points dotted around the body and fine needles are inserted into these points. Acupuncture has been shown to reduce hot flushes in some studies, and the beneficial effect was maintained for several months after treatment. Presently we have, however, too few research studies to be sure.

Reflexology

Reflexology works on the principle of zones whereby the body is divided into areas, and pressure applied to one part can affect another part of the body in the related zone. Usually pressure is applied to the soles of the feet, since the entire body is thought to be represented in parts of the feet. Stimulation of nerve endings in the feet is thought to stimulate the autonomic nervous system and pressure is believed to promote energy flow in different zones. It is not clear exactly how reflexology works, nor if it specifically helps menopausal symptoms, but, as with other complementary therapies, time to yourself, if nothing else, is likely to help.

Although these techniques may well be helpful in reducing stress, allowing 'time out' and generally achieving improved wellbeing, research on their use specifically for menopausal symptoms is lacking.

11 | Medical problems and the menopause

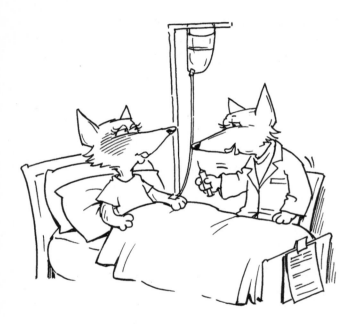

There are many medical problems that can be influenced both by the lack of hormones associated with the menopause, and by the replacement of hormones by HRT. Also, several medical problems may increase the risk of osteoporosis, which should be borne in mind at the menopause and thereafter. Little information is available about the effect of alternative therapies on medical problems. This chapter describes the effect of the menopause and HRT on some common medical problems.

ANGINA

Much controversy continues to surround the topic of heart disease and the use of HRT. It appears increasingly likely that early use of HRT may be protective against heart disease but current opinion states that HRT should not be used solely for the treatment or prevention of coronary heart disease (heart disease). It is also possible that different types, routes and timing of initiation of hormone therapy will have different effects. Menopausal women with angina requiring treatment for menopausal symptoms should be offered non-hormonal therapies initially (see Chapter 9). If these are ineffective and HRT is being considered, women should understand that there is thought to be a small increase in risk of heart attack in the first year of use of systemic HRT in women who already have coronary heart disease. Vaginal oestrogens may be used safely for the treatment of vaginal and bladder symptoms (see Chapter 8).

ANOREXIA

A history of anorexia, particularly if amenorrhoea (absence of periods before the menopause) occurred, increases the risk of osteoporosis (see Chapter 4). This is because being underweight can stop the stimulation of the ovaries from the brain, leading to reduced oestrogen production. The lack of oestrogen at a young age impairs bone strength. The menopause is an ideal time for assessment of risk, and bone density scanning should be considered. HRT can be used for control of menopausal symptoms or prevention/treatment of osteoporosis.

ASTHMA

There does seem to be a relationship between hormones and respiratory function, but the exact association is unclear. Some women do notice a worsening of asthma premenstrually and asthma may improve or worsen around the time of the menopause. The use of HRT may confer a small increased risk of asthma but its use does not seem to worsen pre-existing disease and some studies have suggested a beneficial effect.

BREAST PROBLEMS

Cancer

A history of breast cancer is generally seen as a contraindication to the use of systemic HRT but vaginal oestrogens (see Chapter 8) can be used for the treatment of vaginal and bladder symptoms. For systemic menopausal symptoms (such as flushes), non-HRT therapies (see Chapters 9 and 10) should be offered. Occasionally, if your symptoms are severe and unresponsive to other therapies, HRT may be considered under specialist supervision. A recent trial, the HABITS trial, suggested that HRT may increase the risk of recurrence of breast cancer, but a study in Stockholm showed no increase; the debate continues.

Occasionally, breast cancer treatment causes a premature menopause and an increased risk of osteoporosis. Bone-protective measures should be considered (see Chapter 4).

Cysts

HRT use may be associated with the development of breast cysts. This may deter women with a history of breast cysts from commencing HRT, but this history should not be considered a contraindication.

CERVICAL CANCER

Cervical cancer treatment may cause an early menopause; bone-protective measures should then be considered because of the consequent increased risk of osteoporosis. If menopausal symptoms occur, HRT can be considered since there is no known association between HRT use and cervical cancer.

COELIAC DISEASE

Coeliac disease is thought to cause poor absorption of calcium by the body, and hence reduced bone mineral density with an increased risk of osteoporosis. Bone-protective measures should therefore be considered, particularly at the menopause (see Chapter 4). If you want to take HRT, you will probably be offered patches for more reliable absorption, since oestrogen from tablets may not be absorbed from the bowel very well.

CROHN'S DISEASE

If you have Crohn's disease, you have an increased risk of osteoporosis from long-term steroid use for the condition and HRT will be absorbed poorly. At the time of the menopause, you should be offered a bone assessment and, if you choose to take HRT, you may be given patches to ensure adequate absorption.

DIABETES

Women with type 1 diabetes are thought to be at increased risk of osteoporosis and coronary heart disease. The association between HRT use and diabetes has caused some confusion – some studies show a reduced risk of diabetes in women taking HRT, but recent HRT information sheets from pharmaceutical companies advised caution in diabetic women. Currently, it is thought that HRT may be used when indicated in women with diabetes, and that either low-dose tablets or patches are best. If progestogen is required, dydrogesterone (see Chapter 8) seems least likely to interfere with diabetic control, although further studies are required on the ideal type and route of HRT.

ENDOMETRIOSIS

There is a small risk of reactivation of endometriosis (see Chapter 5) with HRT use and any recurrence of symptoms such as pelvic pain should be reported. If you have had a hysterectomy for endometriosis, your doctor will consider the extent of endometriosis at the time of the operation and choose the HRT most suitable for you. If you have had a premature menopause from having a hysterectomy (see Chapter 5), you will be advised to take HRT until the average age of the menopause (51 years).

HRT after hysterectomy usually consists of oestrogen only. However, if any spots of endometriosis have been left behind, oestrogen may cause stimulation of these deposits and you might be given continuous combined (oestrogen plus daily progestogen) therapy, or tibolone, but there is little research on the effect of different types and duration of therapy. Medical treatment of endometriosis often involves ovarian suppression (which 'switches off' the ovaries and therefore reduces oestrogen production from the ovaries while the treatment is being taken, causing a temporary menopause), which, along with ovarian removal, may increase the risk of osteoporosis.

EPILEPSY

Women with epilepsy may have an increased risk of osteoporosis due to the effect of antiepileptic therapy. Firstly, antiepileptic drugs are thought to increase the breakdown of bone, which may result in lowering of bone density in some people. Secondly, anticonvulsants are thought to interfere with the body's use of vitamin D, essential for calcium absorption; this interference consequently impairs calcium absorption. The risk of osteoporosis is particularly increased if antiepileptic therapy is used in high doses, for long-term therapy and when more than one drug is required.

There can be a problem if you need HRT therapy, as some antiepileptic drugs can increase the rate at which your body gets rid of hormonal therapy by stimulating liver enzymes involved with the breakdown of hormones. Low or standard dose oral HRT may therefore be ineffective and the patch route may be preferred.

St John's wort should be used with caution since drug interactions can occur.

FIBROIDS

Fibroids are benign smooth muscle tumours of the wall of the uterus and their growth is dependent on oestrogen. They tend to shrink after the menopause but this might not happen, or they might even increase in size with HRT use. This can occur in 25% of women on HRT, mainly in the first 6 months of therapy. There is some limited evidence that the patch route but not tablets or tibolone, can cause fibroids to grow. If this happens, you may be advised to have regular examinations, and sometimes ultrasound scans, to monitor the size of the fibroids. There is some evidence that the progestogen-releasing intrauterine system, such as Mirena, may cause fibroids to reduce in size. Mirena is often given to women in the perimenopause who have heavy periods and/or require contraception, and it can provide the progestogen part of their HRT.

GALLBLADDER DISEASE

HRT has been shown to increase the risk of gallbladder disease, particularly gallstones, thought to be due to an effect on the composition of bile; the fluid secreted by the liver, concentrated in the gallbladder and then poured into the small intestine. If the concentration of bile constituents is affected, deposits of salts may occur in the gallbladder, causing gallstones. Increasing age and obesity increase the risk of gallbladder disease and it may be that HRT users who develop problems may have had silent gallbladder problems already, which are worsened by HRT. If you have a history of gallbladder disease, you will probably be offered HRT in patch form.

HYPERLIPIDAEMIA

If you have hyperlipidaemia (high blood fats), this does not mean you cannot take HRT, but your doctor will decide on the best type and route of HRT, since the type and route can have effects on certain lipids. For example, oral oestrogen generally increases triglyceride levels, so the patch route is preferred if you have high triglyceride levels. Oral oestrogen can also, however, lower cholesterol levels, which is a bonus.

HYPERTENSION (HIGH BLOOD PRESSURE)

Before you are offered HRT, your blood pressure will be measured and, if it is high, this will be treated first. You will have further blood pressure measurements at 3 months after starting HRT, and it is then usually checked at an annual review. There is a very small risk of conjugated equine oestrogens (see Chapter 8) causing a rise in blood pressure but this will return to normal once HRT is stopped. If hypertension is already controlled, HRT is unlikely to worsen control; some doctors recommend using non-oral (transdermal such as the patch or gel) HRT.

Take sage with caution if you have high blood pressure and, if you are already taking antihypertensive therapy, take St John's wort also with caution. It is best to tell your doctor what else you are currently taking.

JAUNDICE *(see Liver disease)*

KIDNEY FAILURE/TRANSPLANT *(see Post-transplant; Renal failure)*

LIVER DISEASE

If you have a history of liver disease but your liver function has now returned to normal, you could take HRT, but the non-oral (trans-dermal) route would usually be advised. If your liver disease is still active, and your liver function tests abnormal, you would probably not be prescribed HRT.

MIGRAINE

Migraine is often triggered by hormonal fluctuations and therefore can occur around the time of a period. Such migraine may improve at the time of the menopause. Some women find that migraine can be triggered by the daily hormone fluctuations, which oral HRT can cause, so the patches are probably best if you have a history of migraine. If you are postmenopausal, using a period-free type HRT rather than a monthly bleed type may improve migraine, since there is less fluctuation in the progestogen level.

MELANOMA

For many years, doctors thought that women who had a history of malignant melanoma should not be given HRT but this is now controversial – it is now thought highly unlikely that there is an association between development and progression of melanoma and HRT.

MULTIPLE SCLEROSIS

Menopausal women with multiple sclerosis have additional risk factors for osteoporosis and fracture, namely reduced mobility and ability to do weight-bearing exercise, low levels of vitamin D, sometimes previous courses of steroid treatment and higher likelihood of falling. Women with MS should take bone-protective measures – advice from health professionals and specific treatments (see Chapter 4). HRT can also be taken.

OTOSCLEROSIS

This inherited condition causing progressive deafness has been shown to worsen with pregnancy and, very rarely, with the contraceptive pill, but there is no evidence that HRT has such an association.

OVARIAN CANCER

A history of ovarian cancer is not currently a contraindication to HRT.

PARKINSON'S DISEASE

Some studies have suggested that use of oestrogen after the menopause may reduce the risk of Parkinson's disease and there is certainly no evidence of a worsening effect associated with HRT use.

POST-TRANSPLANT

Women who have had organ or marrow transplants have an increased risk of osteopenia (low bone density) or osteoporosis, thought to be as high as 80%, with osteoporosis-related fracture expected to affect up to 65% of transplant patients. Post-transplant steroid and other immunosuppressive therapy is thought to play a part in the bone loss, as well as the illness leading to the transplant, and its treatment, often causing an early menopause. Such women should consider taking HRT and other bone-protective treatments.

RENAL FAILURE

Renal failure increases the risk of early menopause, and osteoporosis. Although HRT and other bone-protective treatments can be taken, little information exists about benefits and risks in such women.

RENAL TRANSPLANT *(see Post-transplant)*

RHEUMATOID ARTHRITIS

Rheumatoid arthritis (RA) confers an increased risk of osteoporosis, thought to be related to steroid therapy, increased bone resorption and reduced ability for weight-bearing exercise. Women with RA should consider using HRT or other bone-protective measures. HRT does not appear to affect disease progress.

STROKE

The incidence of stroke increases in women after the menopause. Ovarian hormones, oestrogen and progesterone, possibly protect women before this time. Similarly, it was thought that HRT reduced the risk of stroke. Although some studies have shown a protective effect, others, including the Women's Health Initiative trial, have shown a small increase in risk of stroke in those women taking HRT. However, a more recent study reported from Sweden of almost 17,000 women aged 45–73 years, showed no significant association between hormone use and risk of stroke. At the moment, it is recommended that HRT should not be used for prevention of stroke. If a woman has had a stroke and is considering treatment for menopausal symptoms, non-hormonal options should be tried first (see Chapters 9 and 10), and HRT should be considered only after full discussion with a specialist.

SYSTEMIC LUPUS ERYTHEMATOSUS

Systemic lupus erythematosus (SLE) is a multisystem disease that can cause rashes, seizures, kidney problems, blood disorders, fever, pericarditis (inflammation of the pericardium, the fibrous membrane around the heart) and arthritis. Women with SLE are at increased risk of osteoporosis because of steroid therapy. Although SLE is thought to be linked to hormonal levels, and indeed often worsens during pregnancy, there is no evidence of a worsening effect if HRT is taken. However, SLE may be associated with venous thrombosis in which case HRT should be used cautiously.

THROMBOSIS

Since HRT is associated with a small increased risk of *venous thrombosis*, women with a past history of thrombosis will be given advice on the risk factors if they want to take HRT. Depending on why HRT should be given and on the cause of the thrombosis, risks and benefits will be assessed. If HRT is given, it will normally be via patches. All women with thrombosis should seek specialist advice. Vaginal oestrogen may be used for the treatment of vaginal and bladder symptoms.

THYROID DISEASE

Hyperthyroidism, from either an overactive thyroid gland or over-replacement of thyroxine in underactive thyroid disease, leads to an increased risk of osteoporosis because of excess bone loss – raised thyroid hormone levels have an effect on the activity of both osteoblasts and osteoclasts, with a predominant effect on osteoclasts, and this leads to increased bone resorption (see Chapter 4).

Postmenopausal women who have a history of hyperthyroidism should be screened for osteoporosis and offered bone-protective measures. HRT does not worsen thyroid disease and, in fact, may be particularly helpful because of its bone-protective effect. However, if you are taking thyroxine, your thyroid function will be rechecked 3 months after starting HRT because the thyroxine dose may need to be adjusted. Similarly, your need for thyroxine may alter if HRT is stopped, and your thyroid function should be rechecked 3 months after stopping HRT.

UTERINE CANCER

If you have a past history of uterine (womb) cancer, you will not normally be allowed to take HRT. However, if your cancer was of a very early stage and your menopausal symptoms were such that HRT would be useful, your specialist might allow it. Progestogens or other non-HRT therapies could be used as an alternative to HRT for vasomotor symptoms.

12 | Sex, relationships and work

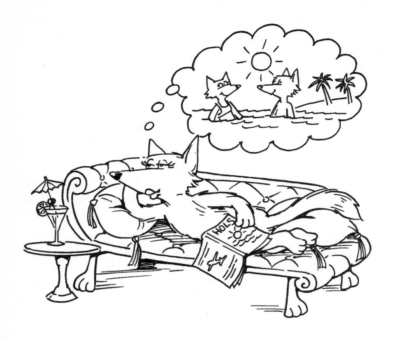

The menopause can affect female sexuality and relationships by various means and sexual problems often occur both with the menopause and with ageing. Sexual problems are estimated to occur in 50% of sexually active women in middle age, yet many women do not disclose the problem. Despite our society being much more open and able to discuss sensitive issues than ever before, many women are still too embarrassed to seek help when things are not quite right. Although some women do not feel that an active sex life is vital, often quoting that they'd rather have a cup of tea (!), 79% of women in a recent survey feel that it is important to continue an active sex life into old age. Since men generally rate sexuality highly as an important quality of life issue, sexual problems often cause relationship problems, while relationship problems may contribute to sexual problems.

Problems can occur from lack of interest or desire, decreased arousal and response and discomfort. Changes associated with the menopause and changes associated with the stage of life rather than hormone changes can all play a part in sexual difficulties at the menopause.

I think I'm going through the change with periods all over the place, hot flushes and sweats. These things I can cope with and was expecting but what has really upset me is the loss of sex drive. My husband and I are very close and he's very understanding but it is putting a strain on our relationship – I can't seem to get him to understand that it's not his fault. Will my sex drive come back or is this it?

Many factors contribute to the common problem of reduced libido or sex drive. Factors that particularly affect menopausal women include sleep disturbance leading to tiredness, nuisance of heavy and irregular periods, tension with partner (which then leads to a vicious circle with reduced sexual activity often causing more tension), stress over other life events (which often happen around the time of the menopause – problems with teenage children, children leaving home, elderly parents, work pressures), menopausal symptoms signifying the ageing process and the need to come to terms with this, and hormone changes affecting response.

The hormones, oestrogen, progesterone and androgens, are all important in sexual desire and response; both oestrogen and progesterone levels fall at the menopause and androgens fall with age, declining particularly after the age of 40 years. The fall in oestrogen may also cause vaginal dryness and discomfort and this can affect desire and response. Because of the role of hormones, some women do benefit from hormone therapy but, for women especially, the other personal and relationship factors are as, if not more, important.

Continued communication with your partner is vital to work through this and find out what is the best option for you. Many women do benefit from some help at this stage, whether it is advice or specific therapy but, with guidance, there is no reason why women can't continue to enjoy an active sex life well into old age!

My periods stopped a few years ago and I was really lucky with the flushes – I only had them now and again for a few months. However, I'm now having pain whenever I have sex with my partner. I'm dry and, to be honest, it puts me off so much that I've started making excuses. I don't want to take HRT because I don't feel I need it but can I take something just for my pain?

The lack of oestrogen causing vaginal dryness and discomfort is a frequent menopausal problem, yet women often don't report it; a recent survey showed that over half (51%) of menopausal and post-menopausal women suffer from bothersome vaginal symptoms, yet the majority of them (79%) had not discussed their symptoms with a healthcare professional. For almost half of these women (47%) these symptoms were so severe that they affected their sex lives. A quarter even said that they make excuses to avoid having sex with their partner.

For vaginal dryness, there are treatments available such as vaginal lubricants and moisturisers, which can be purchased from pharmacies. Vaginal Replens is also now available on prescription. Although you do not want to take HRT, vaginal oestrogen in the form of a small tablet, pessary, cream or vaginal ring is very effective. Because the oestrogen is given in a small dose and is concentrated in the vaginal tissues, very little, if any, of it gets into the rest of your body, and so is not likely to be associated with the risks and side effects of HRT (see Chapter 8).

My HRT has really helped my sweats but has made not a bit of difference to my libido; in fact, if anything, I think it's got worse. Can HRT worsen it or is it my imagination?

Some medicines can cause the body to produce less testosterone, which is important for libido, mood and energy levels. The tablet form of HRT can have this effect, as can the oral contraceptive pill and thyroxine. One type of tablet HRT which does not have this effect is tibolone and in fact tibolone may increase testosterone-like activity production. Tibolone can be considered if your periods have stopped, since it is a 'period-free' preparation. Also, a non-tablet form of HRT, such as a patch or gel, has a lesser effect in reducing testosterone compared with tablet HRT.

THE ROLE OF TESTOSTERONE

Since testosterone (one of a group of hormones known as androgens, produced both from the adrenal gland and the ovaries) is thought to play an important part in sexual interest and response, some women may benefit from testosterone replacement. There is a gradual decline in androgen production with age from the 40s to old age so that, by the time you reach 70, androgen levels are 70–80% less than in earlier years. A 50% reduction in testosterone levels is seen following removal of the ovaries. Symptoms of androgen deficiency include persistent fatigue and low mood as well as the low libido. Testosterone replacement may be considered in women who have had their ovaries removed, and women on tablet HRT who have symptoms suggestive of testosterone insufficiency may wish to try a different route or type of HRT.

Blood levels of testosterone do not seem to bear a close relationship to response and there are currently few testosterone preparations that are licensed for use by women. Apart from the HRT preparation, tibolone, the only other licensed way for women to take testosterone is by an implant. This is a small pellet placed under the skin of the abdomen every 6 months. Testosterone patches and gel are available for men but are being used a little in women in smaller doses. A recent study showed that testosterone gel improved frequency of sexual activity and sexual interest in postmenopausal women taking HRT but the appropriate dose for women has yet to be determined. Therefore the subject of testosterone replacement is still controversial and subject to further research.

Although a change in the type of HRT or, for some women, some form of testosterone along with HRT is worth considering, the many other factors affecting libido should not be ignored.

RELATIONSHIPS

Women often need to feel secure, loved, wanted and emotionally close to their partner to be able to fully enjoy sexual relations. A domestic dispute leading to disagreement can continue to cause disharmony; men can feel that making love allows them to show their love for their partner and make up for the disagreement, whereas women often need to have the disagreement sorted out before they will feel close enough to enjoy a sexual relationship, and hence failure to resolve this different approach causes further tension. (See Fig. 12.1)

The menopausal changes of weight gain, skin changes and impact of loss of fertility can all affect self-confidence in a woman, influencing how she feels about herself, her relationship and her sexuality. On the other hand, she may find that the menopause has a positive effect on sexual response by signalling the end of heavy and often painful periods, negating the need for contraception and allowing more freedom and time with her partner, especially if children have left home.

Sadly, for some couples, children leaving home may highlight relationship problems that have previously been masked by the activities surrounding the children. Some couples find that they have little in common any more and may have to learn to have fun together again without the children. Relationship counselling can be very helpful in this situation. Any relationship difficulties have a huge impact on sexual response.

Sexual difficulties can also be due to medical problems and medications. Sexual problems affect about 30% of men, erectile dysfunction (impotence) being the most common problem. Men are often even more reluctant than women to report problems and seek treatment. As difficulties continue, tension builds up and the problem escalates. Effective treatment is available and medical help should be sought sooner rather than later.

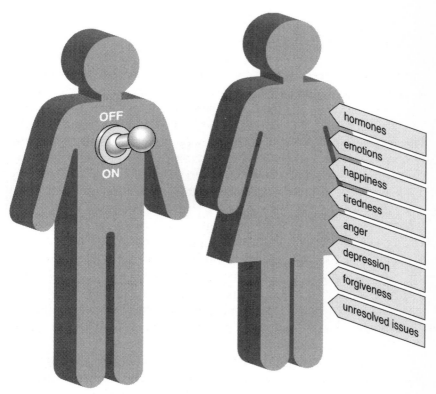

Figure 12.1 Different effects on libido in men and women!

Not just sexual relationships but relationships in general can be affected by the menopause and partners and children often feel confused and don't know how to help.

> *My wife has been going through the menopause for 2.5 years. Her mood swings are getting worse and she is very sensitive to anything remotely personal (comments and such). She had a partial hysterectomy 12 years ago and has only one ovary. We have two kids aged 12 and 9 and they are experiencing hell too. Her memory loss is worsening. She sleeps very little (because of the flushes), and therefore she is tired, which causes her to be more irritable. What I need to know is where should I start in helping her to get control back in her life?*

Being aware of the problem and understanding that it's not her fault is a major help in itself. Explaining this also to your children and just asking them to be patient is very worthwhile. The next step is to help her find information so that she can understand what is happening and know that help is available. This, however, is where diplomacy is absolutely essential because many women do not want to face up to the fact that they are struggling and put off seeking help. Sometimes women see it as a sign of weakness that they can't cope with something that is meant to be natural and that millions of women before them have coped with. Emphasise the fact that you want to help, that you're not being critical, and suggest books (you are obviously already looking at this one!), magazines, or the internet. You could encourage her to make a visit to her doctor. Many women feel better by just knowing that they are not alone and that many women are experiencing the same problems, and by hearing what has worked for others. Support groups are available including the very popular online groups. Once she is aware of what's going on, then lifestyle changes and diet may be relevant, or specific treatments can be considered.

SEXUALLY TRANSMITTED INFECTIONS

With divorce rates increasing all the time, menopausal women may find themselves in new relationships. Older people are not generally thought to be at risk of sexually transmitted infections (STIs) but, in fact, for several reasons, they may be at higher risk and treatment may be delayed owing to a lack of awareness of the problem.

In women aged between 45 and 60 years in the UK in 1995–2003, reported rates of syphilis increased by 275%, chlamydia by 175% and gonorrhoea by 254%, yet most educational prevention programmes continue to be directed at younger people.

After being on my own for 6 years, I am now in a new relationship. I've not had a period for about 3 years so I know I don't need to use contraception but should I suggest to him that we use condoms?

One of the reasons that menopausal women are at increased risk of sexually transmitted infections is that, since they often don't need contraception, they may think that there's no reason for barrier contraceptives, and they have unprotected sexual intercourse. In fact condoms are an excellent method of reducing the risk of infection and should therefore be used in a new relationship even if not for contraception.

The lack of oestrogen as a result of the menopause can cause reductions in secretions of the vagina, change in acidity and thinning of the vaginal tissues, which, together with the age-related decline in immune function, can lead to an increased risk of sexually transmitted infections including HIV. As you are in a new relationship, it is important to be aware of this possibility, so use protective measures even if contraception is not required and report any problems such as vaginal discharge, pelvic pain, discomfort during intercourse, irregular bleeding or bleeding after intercourse. These symptoms are often thought to be due to menopausal or other gynaecological changes, and STIs can be missed if you or your doctor are not aware of the possibility in your age group.

Indeed, delay in reporting symptoms has been noted – more than 40% of women over the age of 50 with an STI in one study waited 2 weeks or more before seeing their doctor, because of lack of awareness; they did not appreciate that they may be at risk, and they were also embarrassed. The majority of participants in a study reported in 2001 stated that they had not received much information on STIs or HIV. The advice regarding safe sex is generally targeted towards the younger generation, but menopausal women are particularly at risk of STIs and both they and their health professionals should be alerted to this possibility.

WORK

Women's role in society has changed dramatically over the last few decades, with many women now having full-time careers and running households at the same time. Despite the introduction of labour-saving devices such as automatic washing machines, tumble dryers, convenience foods and microwaves, working and keeping everything ship-shape at home is no mean task. Although women now have a great involvement in paid work, they are still doing 70% of the housework, and many are still the primary child-rearer. Today's image of the modern superwoman as being able to cope with work, having the house beautiful, producing tasty, nutritious meals, bringing up perfectly behaved, charming children and looking like a film star is totally unrealistic but so often expected. The amazing thing is that, in fact, many women do manage to multitask to perfection and do achieve most of what is expected until menopausal symptoms and concerns appear and tip this delicate balance.

Since I hit the menopause, I just can't cope anymore – I can't do all the things that I managed to fit in before without any bother. I see my friends rushing around working, their houses always looking like something from Ideal Home, and they can produce dinner for 6 at the end of the week. I just want to curl up in front of the TV after work on a Friday night, I'm so exhausted. I feel such a failure. My husband has been really patient but he's getting fed up with me now. I don't want to be like this but I don't know where to start to get help.

The first step in getting through this is accepting that there is a problem; many women find it hard to talk about such feelings because it is often seen as admitting a weakness. Women have such high expectations of themselves and it can be hard to face up to the fact that we can't be superwoman all the time! Explain exactly how you feel to your husband and take a good look at what your week is taken up with. Ask yourself:

- Are there tasks that other people can help with?

- Are there tasks that don't really need to be done at all?

- Is the world going to end if the dust gathers on the mantelpiece?

- Will it matter if Victoria doesn't have a home-made cake for her party or if James doesn't have the cleanest football or rugby kit at the start of the match?

Are you having menopausal symptoms such as poor sleeping, flushes and sweats, which some treatment could help? If so, discuss these with your doctor. Think about how you want to spend your time, not how others expect you to spend your time, and make sure that you do something for yourself. Don't compare yourself with others – others are often not really as organised and perfect as they may seem.

The evening after writing this section, having spent all that day working at my computer, I became very grumpy and cross with myself. The reason? I failed to produce the wonderful wholesome Sunday tea that I felt my family deserved and we had pasta instead.

Despite the expectation being totally unrealistic, I still became stressed and grumpy because, in my eyes, I had indeed failed. My family were perfectly happy with pasta, needless to say! It can be difficult to break away from a few decades of setting ourselves these high standards, but stress can be reduced by doing so.

> *Can I keep taking HRT until I retire? It has been a godsend for me. I could hardly get through the day before I started taking it – I was flushing in front of people in meetings, mostly men so it was so embarrassing, and I was so tired through not sleeping that one day I almost fell asleep on my way home. Now that I'm taking HRT, I'm fine again and I couldn't bear to go back to that.*

When HRT is taken for control of menopausal symptoms after the age of 50, current advice is to have a trial off treatment every 2 years or so to see if it is still needed, but many women choose to continue taking it until they retire and life is less busy. At that time, reduction in stress and having more time to relax may mean that symptoms, if still present, are less troublesome and more manageable. If you stop treatment before then, try choosing a time when things are not so hectic if possible. As long as you understand the pros and cons of continuing HRT, then you should be able to choose how long to take it (see Chapter 8).

> *I have struggled with the memory loss aspect of menopause, as I have always been notorious for my ability to remember everything. Now, I can remember things from way back but constantly forget something my boss asked me to do only the day before. Have you any tips to help me?*

Write everything down in a notebook and make sure that you really focus on what you are being asked to do and what people say to you. Using simple tips like this or making lists to cope with problems such as memory changes can help greatly.

Balancing work and home life can be challenging at any age but can be particularly difficult with the onset of menopausal symptoms. Be prepared to explain to your family how you are feeling and don't be frightened to ask for their help. They may be used to you doing everything for them but would be very happy to help more if they knew that you were struggling.

The menopause is often a time of life when women are well established in the work place and taking on extra responsibilities. This, coinciding with problems with worrisome teenage children and elderly relatives, is a recipe for extreme stress, which, in itself, can worsen symptoms and affect coping abilities.

Of course there is no single solution to the 21st-century problem of busy stressed people but some simple principles can provide some help and are particularly relevant at the menopause.

- Taking time to decide what is most important is essential – only you can decide what is really important for you and your family and, once you have decided, then you can take measures to prioritise.

- Make time for yourself to do something that you enjoy – it doesn't matter what it is. This may be the first time in many years that you have so 'indulged' but it is important to be you, not always wife, mother, work colleague, daughter.

- When at work, make sure that you eat healthily and regularly and take a proper lunch break. Many women skip lunch. Eating irregularly and poorly may exacerbate the menopausal symptoms of tiredness, poor concentration and irritability. Getting away from your work place, even just for a short break, can aid concentration.

- Don't be frightened to delegate both at work and at home; accept that you can't do everything all the time.

- Exercise has undoubted benefits, not only for health around the menopause, but general health also. Working women may find difficulty fitting in an exercise programme to their busy schedule but making it a priority is well worth the time investment. Simple tips for starters include parking in the furthest away corner of the car park, walking to work if possible, taking the stairs instead of the lift and going to a higher floor than you need to.

- Changes in body appearance and self-image at the menopause can lead to lack of confidence, especially if you are working with young beautiful people, Be confident that your experience of life, maturity and wisdom has much to offer in the work place – don't be undermined by young work colleagues who don't have any wrinkles!

- Approach the menopause with a positive attitude, knowledge, empowerment and confidence. However it affects you, it should not impair your quality of life. Take control, whether it is by lifestyle changes, medication or complementary measures. Know that help is available when necessary and live as full a life as possible.

Glossary

atrophy reduction in size or thinning of a structure.

autoimmune disorder a disorder in which the body produces antibodies (normally produced as part of the defence mechanism, e.g. against infection), which work against our own organs.

bone remodelling reorganisation of the structure of bone by the effects of osteoclasts and osteoblasts.

climacteric the transition from normally functioning ovaries to the end of ovarian function.

collagen main supportive protein of skin, tendon, bone and cartilage.

coronary heart disease disease of the coronary arteries, which supply blood to the heart muscle.

corpus luteum the area of the ovary which produces progesterone after egg release.

densitometry determination of the density of a material.

dual energy X-ray absorptiometry (DEXA) scan a type of X-ray that determines the density of bone and from which osteoporosis is diagnosed.

endometrium the lining of the womb stimulated by the ovarian hormones through cycles of thickening and then shed.

endometriosis the presence of cells of the endometrium outside the womb.

follicle stimulating hormone (FSH) one of the hormones produced by the pituitary gland, which stimulates egg development in the ovary and which rises as ovarian function decreases.

hysterectomy removal of the womb.

idiopathic osteoporosis osteoporosis without a known cause.

inhibin a hormone produced from the ovary that inhibits the production of FSH.

kyphosis abnormally increased curvature of the thoracic spine.

libido sexual desire.

luteinising hormone (LH) hormone produced from the pituitary gland, which stimulates ovulation; egg release from the ovary.

menstrual cycle the cycle of egg development and release, with consequent release of hormones, which stimulate the womb lining and result in shedding of the lining (periods) in the absence of pregnancy.

menstruation the cyclic shedding of the womb lining and bleeding (periods), which occurs approximately 4 weekly during the reproductive years.

oestrogen the main female sex hormone produced by the ovary, spelled as 'estrogen' in the USA and more recently in the UK also.

omega fatty acids a form of polyunsaturated fats, one of four basic types of fat that the body derives from food (cholesterol, saturated fat, and monounsaturated fat are the others).

oocyte egg cells present in maximum numbers before birth and which gradually decline in both number and quality up to the menopause.

oophorectomy removal of the ovary by an operation.

osteoblasts bone cells that build new bone.

osteoclasts bone cells that break down bone.

osteoporosis a disease characterised by thin, fragile bones, with a consequent increase in susceptibility to fracture.

ovaries female reproductive organ producing eggs and hormones, mainly oestrogen and progesterone.

ovulation release of an egg cell from the ovary.

pituitary gland a pea-sized gland situated at the base of the brain, which controls function of other glands, including the ovaries, thyroid, and adrenal gland, also affects growth, milk production, skin pigmentation and water balance by the production of hormones.

placebo an inactive substance used in trials to determine the effect of substances.

premenstrual syndrome cyclical symptoms associated with changes brought about with hormone fluctuations of the ovarian cycle.

progesterone female sex hormone produced by the ovary following egg release.

saturated fat fats can be classed as either saturated, monounsaturated or polyunsaturated, depending on the type of chemical bonds present. Saturated fats tend to be animal fats, such as butter, lard, suet and meat, and are solid at room temperature. Unsaturated fats are liquid at room temperature. They are usually of plant origin, though fish oils may also be high in polyunsaturated fatty acids.

surgical menopause menopause caused by removal of the ovaries by operation.

vasomotor symptoms symptoms of hot flushes and sweats caused by altered function of skin blood vessels and sweat glands.

venous thrombosis blood clot causing blockage of a vein.

Appendix 1 – Useful addresses and websites

Menopause Matters Ltd
Website: www.menopausematters.co.uk
Founded and managed by Dr Heather Currie, Menopause Matters runs the independent, clinician-led Website www.menopausematters.co.uk and publishes the quarterly Menopause Matters *magazine.*
Dumfries-based helpline:
01387 241121
Run by a Menopause Nurse specialist: Thursdays 9am–12 noon.
Gives advice/information about menopausal queries, HRT, alternatives and osteoporosis.

British Acupuncture Council
63 Jeddo Road
London W12 9HQ
Tel: 020 8735 0400
Website: www.acupuncture.org.uk
Provides information for professionals and the public. The Website has an online search facility to enable you to find an acupuncturist in your area.

British Association for Counselling and Psychotherapy
BACP House
35–37 Albert Street
Rugby CV21 2SG
Helpline: 0870 443 5252
Website: www.www.bacp.co.uk
Publishes a directory of qualified counsellors and psychotherapists.

British Complementary Medicine Association
PO Box 5122
Bournemouth BH8 0NG
Tel: 0845 345 5977
Website: www.bcma.co.uk
The BCMA is a professional body which supports the integrity of its therapists and ensures the protection and wellbeing of their clients.

British Herbal Medicine Association
1 Wickham Road
Boscombe
Bournemouth BH7 6JX
Tel: 01202 433691
Website: www.bhma.info
Publishes relevant reading matter and provides information about qualified herbal practitioners.

British Holistic Medical Association
PO Box 371
Bridgewater
Somerset TA6 9BG
Tel: 01278 722000
Website: **www.bhma.org**
Provides information about the principles of holistic medicine; publishes a directory of members and a list of books and tapes.

British Homeopathic Association
Hahnemann House
29 Park Street West
Luton LU1 3BE
Tel: 0870 444 3950
Website: www.trusthomeopathy.org
Provides an information service, a book list and newsletter, and details of registered practitioners.

British Menopause Society
4–6 Eton Place
Marlow
Bucks SL7 2QA
Tel: 01628 890199
Website: **www.the-bms.org**
A registered charity dedicated to increasing awareness of post-menopausal healthcare issues and promoting optimal management through conferences, roadshows and publications.

Daisy Network
PO Box 392
High Wycombe
Bucks HP15 7SH
Website: www.daisynetwork.org.uk
A registered charity for women suffering from premature menopause.

Institute for Complementary Medicine
PO Box 194
London SE16 7QZ
Tel: 020 7237 5165
Website: www.i-c-m.org.uk
Provides advice about how to find registered practitioners in your area.

Institute of Optimum Nutrition
Avalon House
72 Lower Mortlake Road
Richmond
Surrey TW9 2JY
Tel: 0870 979 1122
Website: www.ion.ac.uk
Provides information, publishes the magazine Optimum Nutrition, *and holds a register of professionally accredited nutritional therapists.*

International Federation of Professional Aromatherapists (IFPA)
82 Ashby Road
Hinckley
Leicestershire LE10 1SN
Tel: 01455 637987
Website: www.ifparoma.org
The IFPA supports the professional development of aromatherapists and provides information for the public. It also holds a Register of Professional Aromatherapists throughout the UK.

International Federation of Reflexologists
78 Eridge Road
Croydon
Surrey CR0 1EF
Tel: 020 8645 9134
Website: www.intfedreflexologists.org
Provides information and book/tape reviews. Phone the head office for information about finding a reflexologist in your area.

National Association for Premenstrual Syndrome (NAPS)
41 Old Road
East Peckham
Kent TN12 5AP
Tel: 0870 777 2178
Helpline: 0870 777 2177
Website: www.pms.org.uk

National Osteoporosis Society
Camerton
Bath BA2 0PS
Tel: 0176 147 1771
Helpline: 0845 450 0230
Website: www.nos.org.uk
Use the Website or office number to obtain NOS publications and Information Sheets. Use the Helpline to contact the NOS osteoporosis nurses or email them on nurses@nos.org.uk. For regular updates on osteoporosis, join the NOS online today at www.nos.org.uk or telephone 01761 473117 or 01761 473119 to speak to one of the Membership Co-ordinators.

Women's Health Concern Ltd
10 Storey's Gate
Westminster
London SW1P 3AY
Nurse counselling service:
0845 123 2319
Website:
www.womens-health-concern.org

Appendix 2 – Useful reading

General

Action Plan for Menopause, by Barbara Bushman and Janice Clark Young. Published by Human Kinetics Europe Ltd.

Could it be Perimenopause? by Steven R. Goldstein and Laurie Ashner. Published by Vermilion.

Is it Me or Is It Hot in Here? by Jennie Murray. Published by Vermilion.

The Menopause Bible: The complete practical guide to managing your menopause, edited by Robin N. Philips. Published by Carroll and Brown.

The Menopause – What You Need to Know, by Dr Margaret Rees, Prof David Purdie and Dr Sally Hope. Published by The British Menopause Society and Royal Society of Medicine Publications.

Menopause: The complete guide to maintaining health and wellbeing and managing your life, by Dr Miriam Stoppard. Published by Dorling Kindersley.

The Premature Menopause Book: When the 'change of life' comes too early, by Kathryn Petras. Published by Avon Books.

Your Change, Your Choice, by Michael Dooley and Sarah Stacey. Published by Hodder Moribus.

Alternative therapy

The New Natural Alternatives to HRT, by Marilyn Glenville PhD. Published by Kyle Cathie.

Know Your Complementary Therapies, by Eileen Inge Herzberg. Published by Age Concern Books.

The Phyto Factor: A revolutionary way to boost overall health and control the menopause naturally, by Maryon Stewart. Published by Vermilion.

Dietary help

McCance and Widdowson's The Composition of Foods: Summary edition, produced by The Food Standards Agency. Published by The Royal Society of Chemistry.

Eat Your Way Through the Menopause, by Marilyn Glenville PhD. Published by Kyle Cathie.

Healthy Eating For the Menopause, by Marilyn Glenville and Lewis Esson. Published by Kyle Cathie.

Natural Menopause, by Dr Miriam Stoppard. Published by Dorling Kindersley.

Loving relationships

Making Love the Way We Used to . . . or Better, by Alan M. Altman and Laurie Ashner. Published by Contemporary Books.

Intimate Relations, by Dr Sarah Brewer. Published by Age Concern Books.

Osteoporosis

Osteoporosis: the 'at your fingertips' guide, by Dr Stefan Cembrowicz and Dr Theresa Allain. Published by Class Publishing.

Index

Page numbers in *italics* indicate a figure or table. Those followed by g indicate an entry in the Glossary.

Have you found **Menopause: Answers at your fingertips** useful and practical? If so, you may be interested in other books from Class Publishing.

HIGH BLOOD PRESSURE
Answers at your fingertips £14.99

Dr Julian Tudor Hart with Dr Tom Fahey

The authors use all their years of experience as blood pressure experts to answer your questions on high blood pressure.

> *'Readable and comprehensive information.'*
> Dr Sylvia McLaughlan,
> former Director General,
> The Stroke Association

BEATING DEPRESSION . £17.99

Dr Stefan Cembrowicz and Dr Dorcas Kingham

Depression is one of most common illnesses in the world – affecting up to one in four people at some time in their lives. *Beating Depression* shows sufferers and their families that they are not alone, and offers tried and tested techniques for overcoming depression.

> *'A sympathetic and understanding guide.'*
> Marjorie Wallace,
> Chief Executive, SANE

OSTEOPOROSIS
Answers at your fingertips £14.99

Dr Stefan Cembrowicz and Dr Theresa Allain

This invaluable guide answers hundreds of questions from people with osteoporosis and their families. With positive, practical advice on every aspect of osteoporosis, this is an essential handbook for people suffering from this common condition.

> *'. . . this easy-to-read book provides us all with an unbiased way to take a positive step towards better bone health.'*
> Dr Miriam Stoppard,
> National Osteoporosis Society Patron

THE BACK PAIN BOOK £17.99

Mike Hage

Nearly two-thirds of adults in the UK have had experience of back pain. Now there's hope – and help – for the sufferer. Instead of addressing specific medical diagnoses, the book offers guidance on how to use posture and movement to ease, relieve and prevent back pain.

> *'The book is the most comprehensive book I have come across as a self-help guide to back problems.'*
> Richard Perry, London

MIGRAINE
Answers at your fingertips £14.99

Dr Manuela Fontebasso

Written by an experienced GP with a special interest in headache and migraine, this book acknowledges the uniqueness of every sufferer's experience. Communication between patient and professional is crucial if this complex condition is to be addressed and the best treatment prescribed.

Reading this book will help you understand the nature of your headache, and will give you the confidence to be involved in all areas of decision-making.

HEART HEALTH
Answers at your fingertips £14.99

Dr Graham Jackson

This practical handbook, written by a leading cardiologist, answers all your questions about heart conditions. It tells you all about you and your heart; how to keep your heart healthy, or, if it has been affected by heart disease, how to make it as strong as possible.

> *'Those readers who want to know more about the various treatments for heart disease will be much enlightened.'*
> Dr James Le Fanu, *The Daily Telegraph*

PRIORITY ORDER FORM

Cut out or photocopy this form and send it (post free in the UK) to:

Class Publishing   **Tel: 01256 302 699**
FREEPOST 16705   **Fax: 01256 812 558**
Macmillan Distribution
Basingstoke RG21 6ZZ

Please send me urgently   *Post included*
(tick below)   *price per copy (UK only)*

☐ **Menopause: Answers at your fingertips** (ISBN 1 85959 155 8)   £20.99

☐ **High Blood Pressure: Answers at your fingertips** (ISBN 1 85959 090 X)   £17.99

☐ **Beating Depression** (ISBN 1 85959 150 7)   £20.99

☐ **Osteoporosis: Answers at your fingertips** (ISBN 1 85959 092 6)   £17.99

☐ **The Back Pain Book** (ISBN 1 85959 124 8)   £20.99

☐ **Migraine: Answers at your fingertips** (ISBN 1 85959 149 3)   £17.99

☐ **Heart Health: Answers at your fingertips** (ISBN 1 85959 135 3)   £17.99

TOTAL _____

Easy ways to pay

Cheque: I enclose a cheque payable to Class Publishing for £ _____

Credit card: Please debit my   ☐ Mastercard   ☐ Visa   ☐ Amex   ☐ Switch

Number _____ Expiry date _____

Name _____

My address for delivery is _____

_____

Town _____ County _____ Postcode _____

Telephone number *(in case of query)* _____

Credit card billing address if different from above _____

_____

Town _____ County _____ Postcode _____

Class Publishing's guarantee: remember that if, for any reason, you are not satisfied with these books, we will refund all your money, without any questions asked. Prices and VAT rates may be altered for reasons beyond our control.